A Patient's Perspective:

Living With

Parkinson's Disease

A Patient's Perspective:

Living

With

Parkinson's Disease

or

Don't Rush Me!

I'm Coping As Fast As I Can!

Jon Robert Pierce

Spectrum Communications *Knoxville, Tennessee*

First Edition

Cover design by Lise C. Bender.
Publishing services by Spectrum Communications
P.O. Box 52721
Knoxville, Tennessee 37950-2721

Library of Congress Catalog Card Number: 89-063189

Inquiries should be addressed to:

Jon Robert Pierce

Parkinsonian

P.O. Box 3204

Oak Ridge, Tennessee 37832

I have written this book based entirely on my own experiences, knowledge and study, and discussions with medical personnel and other Parkinsonians. I hope that what I have to say may be of benefit to the P/D patient, caregiver and concerned families as a supplement to the advice and treatment prescribed by health professionals.

I am not an expert or a professional in the field of medicine. Therefore, I do not want the reader to consider anything I've written in this book as being more than the advice of a friend who has lived successfully for over 15 years with the day-to-day realities of Parkinson's disease.

Keep on coping!

Jon Robert Pierce

Jon Robert Pierce
Oak Ridge, Tennessee
October, 1989

DUM SPIRO, SPERO
(While I breathe, I hope)

To the memory of those Parkinsonians who fought the good fight and, by their example, gave me hope. To my favorite person, my wife Jane, and to Laura Powers, M.D., who first suggested that I write this book.

FOREWORD

Throughout this book, the reader will note that I have consistently referred to the Parkinson's disease patient as he, his or him. The only significance of this terminology is that the forms "he or she" or "he and/or she" are so clumsy that, at the risk of being called chauvinistic, I have chosen the shorter form.

The population figures for persons with Parkinson's disease would seem to indicate that the disease occurs more frequently in women than in men. It should be remembered, however, that in the age groups of 65 and older -- the age group where Parkinson's disease is most frequently found -- women outnumber men by a ratio of about three to two. Allowing for this discrepancy it appears that any difference between the number of men and women with P/D is statistically insignificant.

It will also become evident that I have written about the P/D patient as a team with his spouse. This is deliberate. I have often said, only half joking, that my advice concerning Parkinson's disease is, "In the first place, don't get it. If you do get it make sure that you have a loving and understanding partner." The P/D patients who are coping best with their disease invariably have the full and cheerful cooperation of a loving spouse, a caring relative or a dear friend.

How to avoid feeling alone is one of the very real problems discussed later in this book.

A Crash Course for the Parkinsonian in a Hurry

Parkinson's disease:

is bad. Don't get it.
is bad. There are things that are worse.
is progressive but slow.
is irreversible but not life threatening.
is disabling but not overnight.
is incurable but treatable.
is being studied but basic research is slow.

Parkinson's disease:

has good available medication, not perfect.
has few prohibitions but many limitations.
means exercise was important before, vital now.
means dietary rules are not restrictive.
affects muscles. The brain has none.
means mental health lasts though the body weakens.

Parkinson's disease:

patients should stay aware. Don't become a bore.
patients should bc involved. Support groups need workers.
patients should keep a positive attitude.
patients should bless the cheerful caregiver.
patients should be realistic about your limitations.
patients should enjoy life! Good before, better now.
patients should enjoy loose clothes, comfortable shoes.

Parkinson's disease:

If you are smiling broadly at all of this you are a well-adjusted Parkinsonian -- or you don't have the disease.

Table of Contents

Introduction..1-6

About the Author, 1
About the Copilot, 1
About the Subtitle, 2
About the Caregiver, 3
Terminology, 4

What Is Parkinson's Disease?....................7-14

Incidence and Symptoms, 7
Treatment, 9
Connection to Encephalitis........................ 9
A Surgical Procedure and a Chemical Revolution....10
Advances in the 80s................11
Evaluation Scales, 12

Who Gets Parkinson's Disease.................15-19

Research Findings and Theories, 15
Unfounded Fears and Life Expectancy, 17

Why Me?.. 20

Who Diagnoses Parkinson's Disease?.....21-26

Making the Diagnoses, 22
Telltale Signs, 23
Salivation defects...............23
Speech difficulties...............24
Tendency to fall...............24
Suceptibility to hot and cold...............25
Doctor/Patient Relationships, 25

What The Doctor Forgot To Tell You..........27-31

Advance Preparations, 28
Symptoms Present vs. Symptoms Future, 29
Bilateral or Unilateral, 30
Loss of dexterity...............30
Bruxism...............31

Things To Take Heart About......................32-35

A Bonus Of Time..36-41

Breakthroughs in Research, 37

Psychological Effects...............................42-45

Overcoming Depression, 43

Psychological Coping...............................46-53

Recognizing and Coping with Change, 46
Avoiding depression...............48
Negative Attitudes and Misinformation, 51

Physiological Effects................................54-58

Overcoming Physical Difficulties, 55
The threat of falls...............55
Dealing with fatigue...............57

Physiological Coping................................59-64

A Typical Scenario, 59
Bathroom necessities...............61
Morning routine...............62
Bedtime routine...............64
Tips for a More Restful Night, 65

Things No One Will Talk About..................69-76

Sexual Concerns, 70
Dealing with Incontinence, 73

Helpful Hints..77-100

Manual Tasks, 80
Eyesight, 82
Swallowing, Breathing, Speech Difficulties, 84
Teeth and Dental Care, 88
Blood Pressure, 89
Cramps, 90
Diet, Nutrition, Digestion and Elimination, 91
Driving an Automobile, 96
Paraphernalia, 98
Morning Ablutions, 99

Exercises..101-109

Where To Get Help..................................110-115

Getting Help Locally, 111
Addresses for National Groups, 114

Do's AndDon'ts..116-120

For the Patient and Caregiver, 116
For the Caregiver, 118
For the Patient, 119

One Man's Chronology..........................121-127

Postscript..128-129

Appendix..130-142

Parkinson's Incapacity Evaluation, 130
Some of the Symptoms, 132
Useful Medications, 133
Cost of Medication and Treatment, 134
References, 140

Glossary... 143-156

Index...157-160

Introduction

About the Author

Jon Robert Pierce retired in 1984 after more than 30 years of far-ranging travels as a construction manager for engineering firms specializing in metallurgical and chemical processes. He is a pilot of light aircraft and sailplanes, a kayaker, a bicyclist and hiker. He was twice honored by governors of Kentucky with the honorary Commission of Kentucky Colonel.

Jon is a published photographer and he has written for newspapers for more than 20 years, writing on a variety of subjects including travel, food and cooking, general aviation, and, more recently, on Parkinson's disease. Jon is married and has two children and two grandchildren. He and his wife, Jane, are active in their local Parkinson's disease support group where he has served as press secretary for the last five years.

About the Copilot

Mary Jane Cobb Pierce was born in southeast Kansas, where she graduated from high school and worked as a secretary for an attorney, a newspaper, a construction company and an electric utility. She met Jon Pierce in a romantic encounter on a bus during World War II, and traveling became a way of life for Jane after she and Jon were married. The family accompanied Jon on engineering projects, including foreign assignments where Jane tutored the children for four years.

Her appellation as copilot is from the days when Jon was an active pilot. On trips in those days, Jane's contribution to the flight was falling asleep before reaching cruising altitude and not waking up until the tires chirped on landing.

In Jon's struggle with Parkinson's disease, Jane's cooperation and support have been so complete and so beneficial that the term caregiver seems inadequate and copilot is a more descriptive term for the partner relationship of this Parkinsonian couple.

Jane is active in her local Parkinson's disease support group, where she is the current president.

About the Subtitle

Parkinsonians are slow. Let us concede that up front.

If your spouse, caregiver, or friend can do a task in a certain length of time you can count on the Parkinsonian taking two, three or five times as long, and it is possible that he may not be able to do the task at all. Stress or pressure tend to make a Parkinsonian slower and clumsier. To have an impatient "normal" fidget as a Parkinsonian tries to open a door, unlock the car, handle coins or put on a coat only adds to the problem.

To live together comfortably, a Parkinsonian and his spouse need to discuss when to assist and when to stand aside.

Get those peeves and irritations out in the open. The Parkinsonian is well aware that he walks slower, dresses slower and eats slower. Everything he does is frustrating to him. How well he succeeds depends a lot on how well the spouse is able to accommodate to a slower, more deliberate pace of living.

Things to remember: (1) the Parkinsonian is not dawdling to antagonize the caregiver; and (2) the spouse is not demanding that the Parkinsonian function as he did before the onset of the disease. A little reason applied to these frustrations in an open adult discussion will do wonders for all concerned with living with Parkinson's disease.

About the Caregiver

The reader will encounter, throughout this book, the term caregiver. Caregiver is a term that has come into use in recent years in an attempt to find a truly descriptive phrase for the individual, family member or not, who provides a major portion of the care required for an ill person, principally in the home.

The term caregiver is an apt one in its implied sense of a caring relationship, providing a service that is beyond mere financial reward. The Parkinsonian who is lucky enough to have a dedicated spouse for a caregiver is fortunate indeed.

I'm sad to relate, however, that the selfless efforts of many caregivers are not fully appreciated. Their dedication and goodwill too often are answered with acrimony and outright hostility by the patient, if the effort is acknowledged at all.

This negative attitude, found in all too many carereceivers degrades the caregiver effort and often turns a loving, freely provided service into a grudging task, performed out of duty rather than love.

So, a word to the caregiver and the carereceiver alike:

> *Be aware that caregiving in the best sense provides a service which cannot be bought and paid for. The patient should realize and appreciate this fact and, as a responsible adult, should act accordingly. The caregiver, on the other hand, should give only what he can give freely without feeling martyred.*

Care given out of a sense of duty and with animosity is often worse than no care at all. It behooves both parties to examine and discuss their attitudes and motivations in the caregiving process and to come to grips with any problems before the relationship is damaged beyond remedy.

Terminology

The reader will note that I have, throughout this book, used the terms Parkinson's disease, P/D, Parkinsonism and Parkinsonian interchangeably and not always precisely. These terms have precise meanings. In order to avoid any misunderstanding of the terminology that I have used, please read the following definitions (Taber):

Parkinson's disease, Idiopathic: Parkinson's disease with the diagnosis meeting all the tests for Parkinson's disease but for which no cause is established.

Parkinson's disease, Encephalitic: Parkinson's disease with the diagnosis meeting all the tests for Parkinson's disease but in a patient who has had a history of Encephalitis.

Parkinson's Syndrome: A neurological manifestation in which symptoms associated with Parkinson's disease are present but which cannot be reliably diagnosed as Parkinson's disease.

P/D: An abbreviated term for Parkinson's disease.

Parkinsonism: A neurological disorder which meets four criteria of Parkinson's disease: resting tremor; slow or erratic movements; loss of flexibility (especially in the joints); and postural instability. Parkinson's disease is always Parkinsonism; Parkinsonism is not always Parkinson's disease.

Parkinsonism, drug-induced: A type of Parkinsonism which is caused by identifiable drugs sometimes of the neuroleptic family (Thorazine, Compazine, Resperine), which is reversible when the medication is withdrawn. (This category does not include the MPTP designer-drug induced Parkinson's disease which is believed irreversible and which is a nearly perfect analogue to Parkinson's disease.)

Parkinsonian: For the purposes of this text, refers to a person who has been diagnosed and is being treated as a Parkinson's disease patient.

Kinesia: Kinetics (more properly) deals with motion. The Parkinsonian hears many terms which contain "kinesia", all of which deal with how he moves or doesn't move.

Generally, any word containing "kinesia" refers to movement and words containing "brady" refer to slowness.

Akinesia: Loss of voluntary movement.

Bradykinesia: Extremely slow movement.

Dyskinesia: Rapid abnormal involuntary movements.

Acrokinesia: Exaggerated or excessive movements.

Bradyphrenia: Slow thought processes.

What is Parkinson's Disease? 1

Parkinson's disease is an ailment of the human brain and central nervous system. It primarily affects the portions of the brain which control the motor or movement functions of muscles throughout the body. The disease affects, for the most part, men and women in the age group of 50 and older. The disease has been described as progressive, debilitating, and irreversible but treatable. A grim sounding prospect, but read on. There is help to be had.

Incidence and Symptoms

The disease is not thought to be contagious, hereditary or peculiar to any ethnic, national or geographic group. It appears to affect men and women in roughly the same percentages, although the figures require some interpretation since women survive in greater numbers into the P/D age group.

There is also some uncertainty about the total number of patients in the United States with P/D. There are estimates running from 200,000 to 1,000,000, with the most realistic being under 500,000.

The more common symptoms of Parkinson's disease are: (1) stiff joints; (2) slow movements; (3) resting tremor of the hand(s); (4) mask-like, expressionless face; (5) stooped posture; and, (6) stiff, shuffling walk.

For a more complete list of the many ways in which Parkinson's disease manifests itself, see the Appendix in the back of this book.

Parkinson's disease was first recognized as a separate, discrete disease by the man whose name is now synonymous with the disease, Dr. James Parkinson, an English physician. Dr. Parkinson (1755-1824) used the term "Shaking Palsy" in his treatise on the ailment, which he published in 1817.

Medicine appears not to have been Dr. Parkinson's chief interest and he spent most of his productive years in the area of paleontology.

Dr. Parkinson was described as a "free thinker" by contemporaries and it appears his interest in P/D was primarily intellectual. In fact, he probably never saw some of the patients on whom he based his findings. However, the fact that he recognized a connection between and among the many manifestations of the disease was a breakthrough in his day.

Beyond describing the disease and its characteristics and having his name associated with it, Dr. Parkinson appears never to have had any further interest in diagnosing and treating the disease (Advances in neurology, 1984).

Treatment

For over 100 years after P/D was recognized and described there was very little work done on causes and prevention of the disease. However, in the mid-19th century, Jean Charcot, an eminent French neurologist, did some important work in diagnosis and experimented with botanicals, one of which was Belladona.

Connection to Encephalitis

There was a brief glimmer of hope for the P/D patient during the World War I period, 1917 to 1919, when there was a pandemic outbreak of Influenza, caused by a virus which was named Type A Encephalitis. This viral scourge killed millions all over the world. In addition, it also left behind as a legacy a disease called Encephalitis Lethargica, or Sleeping Sickness, which produced many symptoms also found in Parkinson's disease.

It was thought at the time and into the 1920s that the conditions were related, the supposition being that P/D was caused by a virus. This assumption provided a focus for P/D research which eventually led to the conclusion that the viral hypothesis was either incorrect or could not be proved. The lack of success of that brief period in the 1920s was followed by a period of neglect which lasted into the 1940s with little research conducted on P/D. During this hiatus, there were continued brief flirtations with herbs and botanicals and there was valuable work done on the physical care of the survivors of the Encephalitis Lethargica outbreak. Also, in the Orient acupuncture was tried as a measure to reduce the symptoms of P/D, but with no apparent success (Margotta, 1968).

A Surgical Procedure and a Chemical Revolution

There was a brief flurry of excitement in the post-WWII period when stereotaxic surgical procedures such as chemopallidectomy were being tried to reduce tremor, the most common symptom of P/D. This invasive procedure was based on the presumption of the time that the way to reduce tremor associated with P/D was to freeze a portion of the brain called the Globus Pallidus, using injections of absolute alcohol to freeze and destroy the brain cells which caused the tremor. This procedure did reduce tremor but at considerable loss to the patient since he was trading a resting tremor for paralysis. This was not considered to be a good exchange, and the operation was almost entirely discontinued before the next significant events in the treatment of P/D took place.

The next hiatus, which developed after surgery was found not to be a viable treatment for P/D, lasted until the 1960s. As late a 1962, one medical dictionary gave as recommended treatment: "Regulated diet, rest of mind and body, frequent bathing followed by friction, electric treatments and constitutional remedies" (Taber). Not a very promising outlook, but things are different now. There is reason to hope.

The introduction of L-Dopa, a chemical substitute for dopamine, a neuro-transmitter absent or in short supply in the brain of P/D patients changed all that.

With the introduction of L-Dopa came what can only be described as a chemical revolution in the treatment of P/D symptoms. The patient's symptoms were relieved to such an extent that there were occasions when Parkinsonians previously confined to wheelchairs literally got up and walked after taking L-Dopa. The improvements in the quality of life were so dramatic that patients and caregivers ran out of superlatives. Some equated the benefits of L-Dopa with a landing on the moon.

Since the introduction of L-Dopa in the 1960s, succeeding generations of the drug have come into use offering more relief and fewer or less severe side effects for the Parkinson's disease patient. There have been a number of other drugs coming on the market in recent years which have been useful to the physician in treating the symptoms of P/D. Because of the diversity of individual symptoms among P/D patients, the physician often must prescribe several medications to achieve the maximum benefit for the patient. The table, in the Appendix, lists a number of drugs which have been prescribed for, and appear to relieve, some aspect of P/D. It should be noted that this table is not, by any means, a complete listing of drugs available or in use.

During the 1970s, the improvements in medication readily available to the P/D patient obscured, in part, the fact that while symptoms were relieved, the cause, cure and prevention of Parkinson's disease was no closer than before. Token research was directed toward the basic problems of P/D but little was conducted in the way of a coordinated effort. In several foreign countries surgery was still occasionally done despite the lack of success in the past. The entire research effort was hampered by the apparent inability of the research community to produce a dependable "animal model" of the disease, a virtual necessity in most successful research efforts.

Advances in the '80s

In the early 1980s, this dilemma was to take a drastic change. In California, a mishap in the attempt to manufacture a "designer drug" similar to Demerol resulted in disaster for young drug abusers who took the tainted product known as MPTP. Almost overnight these young people were hit with a chemically induced case of Parkinson's disease, well advanced. Though the episode was disastrous and irreversible to the victims, for P/D researchers it provided a chemical agent which produced Parkinson's disease at will with a readily reproducible "animal model" for use in research of the disease.

Evaluation Scales

After a diagnosis has been made and the illness has been confirmed as Parkinson's disease, the physician needs to evaluate the severity of his patient's disease at the start of treatment. This evaluation, or quantification, is then used as a yardstick for comparison of the symptoms at later dates to assess the effectiveness of medication and progress of the disease. This rating is made using any one of several scales for the evaluation of a patient's P/D.

Two of the systems of evaluation are the H & Y (Hoehn & Yahr) and the URSP (Universal Rating Scale for Parkinsonism), neither of which is ideal. The H & Y is a six-increment scale from 0 (no visible signs of P/D) to V (complete disability, unable to function effectively at any level). The H & Y scale does not have enough subdivisions to deal with the progress of the disease quantitatively. For instance, Stage I represents unilateral symptoms while Stage II represents bilateral symptoms.

The URSP scale is a scale of 0 (no discernible disability) to 176 (complete disability), but I find the increments awkward.

For my own status evaluation and amusement, I do two things. First, I keep track of the time it took me to mow my lawn five years ago, how long it took to walk to the newsstand for a paper then and now, and the increasing duration of some of my favorite walks, post and present. This serves to give me a number of points on a scale or curve and though there is no indication that my P/D will behave in a predictable manner, I enjoy the mental exercise.

Using these projected curves I estimate that by 1995 the next day's newspapers will be on the stands before I can get home with the current issue and by the year 2000 when I have finished cutting the grass it will be time to start again.

Second, and on a more serious note, I have devised a 0 to 100 scale for myself, 100 being the state of my health five years before I learned I had Parkinson's disease, and 0 being completely immobile and unable to function on any level. I use a separate scale for mobility, for communications and for cognition, plus a fourth which is the average of the other three.

By my current estimates, I rate 60 for mobility, 60 for communication and 75 for cognition, giving me an average score of 65. I find it very gratifying to be functioning this well more than 15 years after diagnosis. (Though cognitive ability is not a primary concern in P/D it is a factor to be considered.)

The worsening of Parkinson's disease symptoms, in my own experience and with others with whom I have compared notes, does not seem to be a linear decline where there is a predictable loss of capabilities each year. Rather, it seems that the disease progresses through any number of plateau intervals, interspersed with sometimes precipitous declines which can be set off by trauma, stress or uncertainty. One would expect that once a level of competence had been lost it would be gone forever. Again, in my experience, this is not always the case.

Frequently, after the stress, or whatever the anomaly, has passed or has been resolved, there is sometimes an euphoric return to a former higher level plateau. This improvement or recapture of a better mental state allows the patient to circumvent the tremor and deal with other symptoms which have worsened during the stressful period. It cannot be emphasized too highly that, regardless of the patient's physical limitations, it is of the greatest importance that his emotional health be maintained at a high level. One way to ensure good emotional health is through an understanding of the symptoms of P/D, the benefits of medicines being prescribed along with the side effects associated with them. The tables in the Appendix are a good place to start.

Who Gets Parkinson's Disease? 2

Who gets Parkinson's disease?

The stock answer is: elderly people. And, as a general rule, that is the definitive answer. Parkinson's disease is chiefly found or identified in that portion of the population over 50 years of age. Many P/D patients have some symptoms for months or even years before a physician makes the correct assumptions and sets the diagnostic wheels in motion. This is an understandable but unfortunate set of circumstances brought about because P/D in the early stages can masquerade as one of several dozen other ailments, some so innocuous that valuable clues are sometimes overlooked for far too long.

Research Findings and Theories

There has been increased interest in, and research on, P/D in the last 20 years. The primary objective in P/D research, as in any basic research effort, is to try to discover the cause of the disease. However, recent research efforts have found out more about the effects of the disease than about the cause. There is a vast body of information on things that do not cause P/D, arrived at through a long list of research efforts which failed to produce viable results.

Parkinson's disease research has determined that P/D is not usually inherited and any concern about it being contagious has been pretty well laid to rest. P/D seems to cross ethnic lines as easily as it crosses oceans and national boundaries. The ratio of men to women affected is statistically normal. There seems to be no occupational or lifestyle biases.

Despite a connection of P/D-like symptoms in miners digging for manganese, the unfruitful viral hypothesis concerning the WWI era Influenza outbreak and the unfortunate "designer drug" discovery, there has been no hint of a breakthrough in the laboratory. That is not saying there are no promising avenues toward finding a cause for Parkinson's disease. Actually, there are several.

Higher Correlation in Farming Areas

One promising theory is based on a statistical correlation of P/D cases per thousand in urban areas in Canadian cities against similar rural populations. The theory in this study is that a higher incidence of P/D exists in rural populations where extensive crop dusting is carried on. Unfortunately, these results have not been confirmed in a reproducible research effort by other scientists and until confirmation comes the original results are suspect.

Link to Cigarette Smoking

In recent years there have been a number of studies directed toward a theoretical link between P/D and cigarette smoking. One statistical sample which purported to show such a link was later determined not to be representative. It was declared a true linkage did not occur, but rather the lower incidence of P/D among non-smokers was a coincidental reflection of personality traits. Just another proof that theories are easier to postulate than they are to prove.

Unfounded Fears and Life Expectancy

There are several points-of-view extant among those who have been touched by P/D. There is the non-patient group who has seen someone near and dear deteriorate as a result of P/D. Finally, there is the patient with early Parkinson's disease who hopes for a miracle and a reversal of his condition. Then, there is the Parkinsonian with advanced P/D who would be content with only a halt to his worsening symptoms.

For the first group there is the fear, generally unspoken, of the unknown, especially that P/D may be contagious and that he or she may be in danger from the disease while caring for the affected family member. Most family members go through an anxiety period and are not truly at ease with the P/D patient until they learn from their doctor or support group what to expect.

The patient with early P/D may theorize that, if his condition can be alleviated with drugs, a cure should follow close behind. The patient with advanced P/D sees the news of advances in medical research and surgical treatment handled in a sensational manner by the media and then entertains hope that it may, indeed, not be too late for him to be helped.

The emotional need to be encouraged and reassured is universal and natural. It pains the physician and support group members to have to be the bad-news messengers. However, it must be said that, although there is progress in many areas of research, no cure is expected in the foreseeable future. Nor is the ability to halt the progress of the disease expected anytime soon. The prospect then is what this book is all about: living with Parkinson's disease and making the most of it.

For the spouse or caregiver, the fear of contracting Parkinson's disease can be very real but it is not something that should be of major concern. The statistical probability of the patient's spouse contracting P/D is more remote than the possibility of being struck by lightning. The time and effort wasted in unrealistic fears is better spent in a display of compassion for, and understanding of, the very real dilemmas faced by P/D families.

A similar matter-of-fact attitude can and should be adopted by the Parkinson's disease patient and his family about life expectancy. There is a lot of misinformation circulating about P/D and life expectancy. However, little data exists concerning P/D historically. This is due to several factors: (1) a lack of a central repository for medical records; (2) less precise techniques in diagnosing P/D; and, (3) the past tendency to link or misassign P/D to catch all categories in the past.

Presently, statistical methods are much improved, diagnoses are more precise and medication is available to alleviate and relieve the symptoms of Parkinson's disease. This enables the P/D patient to lead a reasonably normal lifestyle and to have the expectation of a near normal life expectancy.

There is an old saw which everyone hears soon after being diagnosed as Parkinsonian:

> "*One doesn't die from Parkinson's disease!*
> *One lives with P/D and dies of other causes.*"

This is as good a thought as I can think of for the Parkinsonian to carry as a motto -- to do all that he can to alleviate and compensate for his P/D while not neglecting other aspects of physical and emotional health care.

Why Me? 3

This is, by design, the shortest chapter in this book.

My approach to living with Parkinson's disease is to maintain a positive attiude toward life in general and toward P/D in particular. The recently diagnosed Parkinsonian cannot afford to waste valuable time and physical and emotional strength in counterproductive soul-searching and recrimination. Living the remainder of one's life to the fullest extent consistent with one's medical condition is a full-time job. So, spare yourself, and others, the self-pity that "Why Me?" question conjures up.

As is discussed in other chapters, there seems to be no common thread tying Parkinson's patients together: no genetic or hereditary relationship, no racial, ethnic, regional, economic or occupational commonality. A negative opinion of one's self-worth or a lack of self-esteem can counteract the best efforts of family and friends and any number of health professionals, all of whom want to see the P/D patient do well in the management of his disease.

It is sometimes a matter of the patient making a conscious decision to consider whether his glass is half full or half empty. A great deal is riding on the patient making a positive choice.

Who Diagnoses Parkinson's Disease? 4

The initial diagnosis of Parkinson's disease is most frequently made by the patient's family physician. Quite often the family physician will undertake the entire diagnosis and treatment. Others, however, will consult with a neurologist -- a physician who has special training, knowledge and accreditation in the treatment of diseases of the central nervous system -- for a second opinion or for help in management of the disease. Diagnosis and treatment, in my opinion, are best handled by a neurologist, working with the family physician who continues to provide primary health care. Eventually, most Parkinsonians do end up seeing a neurologist, being referred by internists, cardiologists, orthopedists, psychiatrists and others.

Occasionally, there is a delay in referral by a primary physician who is not familiar with all the symptoms of P/D, such as in the case of a patient who has the rigidity but no tremor. In my own case, my family physician missed what he later said were obvious clues for more than two years before an observant radiologist, despite his concerns for his ethical position, gave me a push in the right direction by advising me to get myself referred to a neurologist.

Making the Diagnosis

The neurologist, by training and experience, is a logical medical professional to make the diagnosis of Parkinson's disease and, what is more difficult, to confirm the diagnosis. There is no classic case of P/D. Each case presents a different slate of symptoms with most, if not all, of these symptoms being shared by one or more other diseases. The variety of symptoms, manifestations and hints as to the presence of P/D is virtually endless. They include many subtle clues as well as obvious symptoms. In the very early stages of P/D the bothersome clues noticed by the patient may often be ascribed by the physician to other causes.

So, the diagnosis which is easy for the experienced physician becomes, in its confirmation, a convoluted detective story played out with elaborate and costly space age machines. There are tests for brain tumors and epilepsy, and for past history of injury or trauma. EEG, various brain scans, CAT and MRI, are brought into play to prevent overlooking another ailment masquerading as P/D.

The first clue in my own detective story was my handwriting. Previously, my handwriting had been a fluid, normal-sized script with a decided backhand slope (I am left-handed). Over a period of years it had become smaller, cramped, less legible and laborious.

At the end of two years my writing had almost become a thing of the past. I complained to my family doctor and he blamed it on arthritis from an old elbow fracture. Even peculiar traces in an EKG during a routine examination didn't alert my family doctor. I am truly grateful to that radiologist who made the connection that finally got me to a neurologist.

Telltale signs

To the neurologist I saw that day over 15 years ago diagnosing my disease may have seemed easy. He checked my reflexes with a hammer, had me walk and turn, button my shirt, pick up a pile of coins, and smile my biggest smile. Then he told me that I had Parkinson's disease and, since I didn't yet know what questions to ask, very little else. He did say the disease was treatable, that it was unilateral and early, but that it would get worse.

It was much later that I learned to identify the more common telltale clues of P/D: resting tremor; slow movements; the lack of expression in the face; the inability to produce more than a slight smile; and, an absent or slowed eyelid blink-rate. There is variation through a wide range of tear production capabilities, from abnormally dry eyes requiring eye drops to profuse and involuntary lachrymation.

Salivation Defects

Saliva becomes a problem, sometimes too much and sometimes too little, going from one extreme of needing a mint in the mouth for moisture to a choking excess caused by altered swallowing capabilities. Involuntary clenching of the jaws and grinding of the teeth, properly called bruxism, can be distracting and damaging to teeth. Also, the muscle disturbance around the mouth can cause uncontrollable pursing or relaxation of the lips and can lead to drooling in advanced stages of P/D.

Speech Difficulties

Speech suffers in a number of ways.

First, there is a loss of muscle tone in the lips making enunciation more difficult. Then, the tongue loses some of its mobility, especially for words containing "th" sounds requiring a tongue thrust which becomes almost impossible. Finally, there is a loss of flexibility of the ribcage and a loss of muscle tone in the diaphragm, both acting to diminish the volume and the velocity of air required for speech.

Some patients develop an unsteady head, experiencing an uncontrollable side-to-side or nodding motion. The movement of hands and arms, legs and feet suffer as the range of movement in joints lessens as the lack of mobility and muscle tone feeds on itself. The walking posture suffers as the back bends, thrusting the head forward and causing the P/D patient to walk with bent knees.

Tendency to Fall

The P/D patient's whole mobility suffers as the disease progresses. Walking with rounded shoulders, a forward thrust head and bent knees and a disturbance of the "righting reflexes" often lead to postural instability and a tendency to fall. Some patients tend to fall forward, others backward; some are unstable in any upright position.

Initiating the motion of walking, making turns and changes of direction may become a difficult or impossible task. One or more walking problems may develop with the most common being festination, an increase in the number of steps taken per minute, increasing constantly as the length of steps decreases until the patient is standing in one spot rapidly shuffling his feet, going nowhere.

Another problem with walking is acrotaxia or loss of motor function in the foot, a condition which causes the great toe to drop when taking a step. This can be an added tripping and falling hazard.

Suceptibility to Hot and Cold

The Parkinsonian is very susceptible to extremes of heat and cold, with cold appearing to be worse because it intensifies the tremor while heat tends to reduce energy. Both susceptibilities appear early and persist. They can, if not recognized, compound the symptoms of P/D normally displayed by the patient.

I have noticed in my own case that I have a pronounced "startle reflex" (as I choose to call it), whereby I am likely to react or recoil strongly if I am spoken to or touched by someone that I am not aware is in my vicinity.

Doctor/Patient Relationships

In the matter of diagnosing and treating Parkinson's disease, quite obviously, not all physicians will bring to the doctor/patient relationship the same amount of expertise, compassion and interest in the patient and his disease. In the same vein, not all doctor/patient relationships are amicable and personalities do clash. The P/D patient should be thankful if his initial choice of a physician is one he can trust with his continuing care.

The ideal relationship should be one of mutual interest and respect, and the patient should have no compunction in seeking a practitioner with whom he can enjoy such a relationship.

What the Doctor Forgot to Tell You 5

There is a limit to the information that a physician can give to a newly diagnosed Parkinsonian in the 30 to 40 minutes usually devoted to a visit to a doctor's office. Here, the practitioner tends to focus on the immediate things such as confirming the diagnosis, making decisions as to what medications to prescribe, in what dosages and at what intervals.

One can't argue with these priorities. They are of primary concern to patient and physician alike. What is regrettable is that the process serves to truncate the information process which is so very important to the patient and his family. The patient is left in the dark about items of importance which may not only affect his emotional health but his physical well-being, things that he not only should know but is entitled to know.

Frequently, the physician neglects this important part of patient care for lack of time. Sometimes he deliberately withholds information, deciding that the patient is better off not knowing. All too often, however, the physician doesn't know what the daily routine of a P/D patient actually entails.

Make Advance Preparations

By seeing the patient and spouse together, subtleties in interpersonal relationships reveal themselves. In such interviews the establishment of better insights are facilitated for the doctor, the patient and the spouse, or caregiver. In short, better medical care is given when the spouse is included in the treatment process.

In order for the patient to get the full benefit from his time with the doctor it is helpful if the patient and spouse prepare, in advance, a list of questions they would like the physician to answer. It is also beneficial if the patient and spouse prepare, in advance, a thorough medical history of the patient, listing illnesses, injuries, surgery, allergies and medication being taken for other complaints. This will make the doctor's task a little easier and will enable him to practice better medicine.

Some questions that the Parkinsonian couple will certainly want to ask the doctor are:

What medication(s) are you prescribing for me?
Is there a generic equivalent?
What benefit should I expect from the medication(s)?
How are they to be taken and when?
What are the most likely side effects?
Could you treat my case effectively without these medications?
Do you contemplate a drug holiday in my case?

Symptoms Present vs. Symptoms Future

Often the patient is needlessly inconvenienced by being misinformed or poorly informed. Virtually all medications useful in Parkinson's disease have one or more side effects which can lead the patient through some real horror stories if he has not been properly briefed. In my own case, I suffered days of violent nausea after taking Artane (trihexyphenidyl) simply because I was not told to take the medicine with food. Many times the patient actually learns about these things from information received at a support group meeting in discussions with other patients and caregivers, and not from the doctor.

Symtpoms present vs. symptoms future are, in the eyes and mind of the Parkinsonian, of vital importance and cannot be emphasized enough. The patient wants, and needs, to know what is in store for him and his spouse. His questions should be anticipated, expected and answered with clarity and specificity. Many physicians choose to deal with the patient only and there are good reasons for this approach, namely the privileged status of the physician-patient relationship, when this is feasible. However, many patients and their doctors find that, for Parkinson's disease patients, better results are obtained when patient and spouse are seen together.

The patient should be told the range of symptoms attributable to his disease so that he will not be surprised at their onset, and so that he can be prepared to deal with what he can control and to live with what he cannot control. In addition, any discussion of Parkinson's disease with a P/D patient should examine in detail the functions of the brain, how motor impulses are generated and transmitted, and how P/D affects these impulses.

Bilateral or Unilateral?

The patient should be told whether his disease is bilateral or unilateral and, if unilateral, which side is most affected. The basic elements of the left brain/right brain relationship should be explained and discussed. The concept of brain hemisphere dominance should be explained and the fact that a hemisphere, for the most part, controls the opposite side of the body. The statistical majority of the general public is right-handed and left-brained. There are any number of facets to this concept of dominance.

There are individuals who write right-handed but who have left foot and left hand preferences in other things. The left-handed phenomenon is being studied by a number of research teams in the fields of neurology, psychology and linguistics with the aim of establishing how dominance is determined.

Loss of Dexterity

The patient needs to have at least a passing acquaintance with muscle groups and functions, of minute and gross movements, and sphincters and buccinators to understand and counterattack the advance of his disease. He should know that there are tremors related to P/D which affect the largest muscles in the body, the quadriceps in the front of the thigh and the tiny orbicularis oculis in the eye. He should be aware that these muscles will deteriorate over time as P/D progresses and should understand that the weakening can be delayed and, in part, counteracted by a conscientious exercise program.

The patient should know that he is going to have handwriting problems and a general loss of dexterity. He should know that he will lose volume and intelligibility in his speech; his eyesight will be affected as changes of focus and adjustments to variations of light intensity are slowed. He can expect to have difficulty in swallowing and must exercise care in eating and drinking to avoid choking. (The caregiver should learn and be prepared to use the Heimlich Maneuver, if needed.)

Bruxism and Incontinence

Many Parkinsonians have a problem with involuntary clenching of jaw muscles and bruxism or grinding one's teeth. This can take place while awake or asleep and is more prevalent during periods of concentration or stress. It can lead to extensive tooth wear and damage.

Incontinence or loss of control of bladder and bowel in varying and unpredictable degrees is experienced by many Parkinsonians and may be from other causes which should be investigated. Also, the loss of hearing acuity is an important complaint of P/D patients and too often is written off as a result of the aging process without sufficient investigation.

Additionally, the Parkinsonian often finds that he becomes more susceptible to extremes of heat and cold, with cold intensifying the tremor and heat contributing to reduced mobility.

Things to Take Heart About 6

After the initial shock of being diagnosed as a Parkinsonian has passed and the patient and his family have had an opportunity to learn something about the disease several things happen.

First, they have come face-to-face with the reality of the diagnosis. The patient has survived the denial of the disease and has dealt, in one way or another, with the "Why me?" syndrome.

Second, the patient has had a chance to look around and see that he is not alone and further, that he is, in a way fortunate. The fact is that P/D is a relatively slow-acting disease and the patient will not be snatched from the bosom of his family before the week's end. He realizes that he can come to grips with his mortality with a little deliberation.

Third, the patient notes with pleasure the relief of symptoms provided by the medication prescribed by his physician. He is better able to take on more physical activity as a result of his improved emotional state and better motor control. The danger here is that after a period of euphoria reality returns and the patient must fight the "Why me?" battle a second or third time. Now, however, the patient finds that by being helped with his disease he can usually help himself. Often this period allows the patient to decide how to handle his work, to deal with the prospect of retirement and to shift gears in his lifestyle, substituting less demanding hobbies and avocations.

Self-education

The P/D patient begins to pay more attention to news items concerning the aging process and to reports concerning Parkinson's disease and related neuro-degenerative diseases. It is a positive sign when the patient is interested enough to make an effort toward educating himself. There is a danger inherent here. The media, in fulfilling their duty to get the latest information into print or on the air, may be doing the public a disservice by sensationalizing every shred of new research data. It is well to recognize that research is going on but one should not expect a cure or reversal of symptoms, not in the foreseeable future.

Preparing for the Future

A reasonable state of mind for the Parkinsonian is to enjoy the relief of symptoms provided by medication while recognizing the certainty of the progress of the disease, in the meantime making timely preparations for worsening conditions to come. Some of the things that the Parkinsonian should have in good order include all of the properly executed documents any other mature adult should have prepared.

An Up-to-date Will

Everyone should have an up-to-date will prepared and his Executor should be kept apprised of family financial matters in enough detail to handle any contingency. This is nothing out of the ordinary and is something we should all be careful about. In addition, the patient should execute a durable Power of Attorney, a document which empowers the spouse (or others) to legally handle the patient's business and personal affairs should the patient become unable to function on his own behalf.

Many people, in good health as well as those with illnesses, are executing a Living Will. This is a document which makes known the wishes of the person making the will in the event of a terminal illness, requesting that no extraordinary measures be used to prolong life. The details of a Living Will and its legality vary among the states and it should be carefully and correctly executed.

Request for Autopsy

One final document that the Parkinsonian is urged to execute is a bequest and request that, after death, an autopsy be performed on his brain to aid in the diagnosis, treatment and research on Parkinson's disease.

The reason the Parkinsonian patient is urged to leave very specific instructions requesting an autopsy of his brain are many, complex and vital. The present research that is under way concerning P/D needs, first of all, to be able to confirm the accuracy of the diagnosis of the living patient. Because P/D is so elusive and so often gives the physician conflicting and erroneous clues, confirming diagnoses is vital. When a comparison can be made of brain tissue with what is known of a patient's occupation, age at onset of P/D and various details of lifestyle (and this process repeated many times over) there is the possibility that this may lead to a computer correlation that can solve the P/D riddle at long last.

The national organizations for Parkinson's disease listed in the chapter "Where to Get Help" are useful in providing information on Living Wills and Brain Autopsy Bequests and requirements in specific states.

A Bonus Of Time 7

The Parkinson's disease patient finds that what has been taken from him in reduced mobility, lost dexterity and lessened confidence in his social skills is disconcerting and irreplaceable. In compensation, he finds that in contrast to the rapid fire resolution of other diseases ending very often in untimely death or disability, Parkinson's disease offers the patient and his family a bonus of time. He can take time to come to a deliberate decision concerning the vital family decisions which must be resolved. He is offered the prospect of many years of life to live practically as he chooses, making suitable allowances for the progress of his disease.

The Parkinsonian can look forward to a rewarding life with a carefree retirement. He has a chance to enjoy his children and to know his grandchildren, to spend quiet hours with a beloved spouse, to spend time on another hobby, or to pursue another vocation. Most importantly, he has an opportunity to come to an understanding with himself, to assess his accomplishments, how he feels about himself, what he is, and to pass that to succeeding generations.

Time is also an ally in the sense that every year a P/D patient lives after diagnosis brings a greater likelihood that the research in progress will produce an improved medicine or a scientific breakthrough which could result in dramatic improvement in the control of Parkinson's disease symptoms.

All of the above can be depended upon to give the Parkinsonian some time and space while he adjusts to his changing lifestyle. It is important to recognize that the patient's mental attitude is vital and that a positive point of view is necessary.

Breakthroughs in Research

In following news reports on the subject of P/D in print and electronic media it seems that most of the coverage is directed toward the more sensational aspects of research, brain cell implants and the MPTP animal model research. However, there is a vast body of work going on which is not considered by the media to be newsworthy, but which promises more immediate relief for the patient who is presently well advanced in the progress of the disease.

In order to understand the importance of these concepts we need to consider the more conventional present-day methods for administering medication for P/D.

In virtually every application of the most frequently prescribed medicines for relief of P/D symptoms, administration is by mouth. Though the directions may vary as to dosage and timing the path that the needed dopamine follows in its journey to the brain is slow and circuitous. Medicine in the form of a tablet or capsule is taken by mouth, usually with water to facilitate swallowing. Safely into the stomach, the tablet or capsule is dissolved and joins the other stomach contents (called chyme) in traveling through the duodenum into the small intestine as part of the ongoing process of assimilation.

The process of assimilation passes the vital components of the medicine into the blood stream where it is transmitted to the brain. How the medicine is extracted and transformed in the brain into the needed dopamine is not yet fully understood. What is known is that this method of delivering dopamine to the areas of the brain where it is needed is very inefficient in two principal ways.

First, the small amount of medication to reach the areas where it is needed as compared to the amount contained in the tablet or capsule is infinitesimal, therefore wasteful and expensive. So, an effort is under way to make the process more efficient.

Second, the duration of the beneficial effects of the appropriate medicine is an average of four to five hours. It is not hard to see why it is difficult to maintain a desired level of dopamine in the brain. In fact, the usual state of a P/D patient is one of change. He can be "on," "off," waiting to "turn on" or expecting to "turn off", in a kind of limbo where the Parkinsonian spends a lot of time. The "turn-off" state can be as dramatic and as inconvenient as the delay in "turning on".

Pump-implant Project

For the Parkinsonian, one of the most promising programs in progress is the pump-implant project. The pump, which is being used experimentally, eliminates a substantial part of the body's delivery process by pumping a stream of liquefied medication in constantly metered, minute quantities directly into the blood stream. These pumps are presently installed in a number of ways, some being surgically implanted in the patient's body.

There is a longer history with these pumps in the treatment of diabetic patients who receive metered amounts of insulin in the blood stream permitting a more precise control and management of their disease. The pump, in its application to P/D, has been used successfully in a pilot project and while it may benefit only a percentage of the P/D population it can be considered another step in the control of the disease.

Animal Models

It is an established fact that, in basic research, in order to study a disease in depth one must be able to duplicate the disease and its symptoms at will. Some research can be carried out in the laboratory "in vitro" literally in laboratory, or glass, dishes. In the study of Parkinson's disease the experimenter, however, needs a study "in vivo", in a living subject. Much basic research is done on animals, mice and monkeys for example. The Rh factor in blood is an example of the lifesaving results of "animal models" in basic research, the Rh referring to the Rhesus monkeys in whom the factor was initially proven.

Basic research in Parkinson's disease was hampered for years by the absence of a reliable "animal model" which could be readily duplicated. This problem was eliminated almost overnight by the development of the MPTP designer drug cases barely a decade ago. MPTP was produced accidentally by an outlaw chemist attempting to make a drug similar to Demerol called MPPP and the tainted product was found to produce almost overnight a full-blown case of advanced P/D. Under laboratory conditions MPTP provided the required animal model needed for research on Parkinson's disease "in vivo". These experiments already have produced some promising results and there is good reason to expect more in the future.

Among those following this course of research are the scientists at the Yerkes Primate Center at Emory University in Atlanta.

Surgical Procedures

Another area of research for which it is too early to assess the results of are surgical procedures being done at several locations around the world in efforts to relieve conditions for P/D patients. This surgery is being done on the premise and knowledge that P/D is caused by the failure of cells in certain areas of the brain to produce the usual adequate amounts of dopamine, a neuro- transmitter which is vital to motor functions of the body.

It is known that the brain is less likely to reject implants of foreign tissue than other organs in the body. It is also known that there are other sources for dopamine in the body. Other than the brain, one potent source of dopamine producing cells is the adrenal glands located with the kidneys. Recent surgical procedures have made the patient the tissue donor as well as the recipient by having his own adrenal tissue removed and then surgically implanted into his brain. In theory, the implanted tissue should retain its dopamine producing capabilities and provide the missing neuro-transmitter, the missing element which caused the P/D.

A number of these cell-implant surgeries have been performed in recent years but the benefit, if any, and the duration of any benefit will require months or years to review and evaluate.

Preliminary results have been varied and positive results have not been reproducible, an important consideration in evaluating experimental success. A matter of concern to researchers is what is called the "placebo effect", a phenomenon which unconsciously leads patients, family members and physicians to perceive benefits because they want and expect to be helped by the procedure or treatment.

The same basic surgery also has been performed using brain tissue cells from aborted human fetuses. This procedure, in theory at least, promises to be a more successful implant than the adrenal cells due to some important biological considerations. The principal problem with this line of research is the very important legal and ethical considerations concerning the use of this particular source of material for implants. Until these considerations are resolved very little can be expected from this line of research.

There are other possibilities for sources of implant tissue from animals such as Sus Scrofa, the domestic hog, already a source for valves in heart surgery.

Psychological Effects 8

There are serious psychological problems to consider in coping with Parkinson's disease. Some problems are the result of biological changes in the patient. However, the great majority of problems experienced by the Parkinsonian are probably related to the drastically altered self-image the patient has of himself when he is faced with the realities of P/D. Almost everyone, including those with no known medical problems, has had intervals when he was depressed. The Parkinsonian is no exception.

With the enormity of the adjustment required in the mental attitudes of both the patient and spouse after the diagnosis of P/D it is natural to go through periods of feeling depressed. If a patient is so inclined and is not challenged in the early stages he can wallow in self-pity and apathy, asking "Why me?" and abdicate without a struggle.

This is wasteful of the energy of both the patient and caregiver, and is generally counterproductive. The patient must be made to see the need for continued mental and physical activity. The mind is like a muscle, use it or lose it.

Good and Bad News

So, on the recreational front there is good news and bad news.

The bad news is that the individual has become a P/D patient, most likely has had to retire, or at least has been forced to lead a more sedentary life. The good news is that one finds one's self with time to select, try and discard any number of activities.

On a personal note, I fall in the adventuresome, short-attention-span category. Before I retired I made a list of things I was interested in but had never found time to investigate properly. Not all of these things were of a cerebral nature but most were. That list filled two pages of a legal size note pad. Now, after nearly five years about half the items are still untouched. A list of "things I would like to know more about" should be maintained by every Parkinsonian. It is a great tool toward the maintenance of good emotional health.

Overcoming Depression

Being depressed is a natural state which can be handled by most adults by means of some kind of activity, some socializing or a diversion. In other words "work it out". But being depressed is not the same thing as depression which is a distinct medical condition with readily identifiable symptoms requiring treatment by a medical professional.

Treatment

Treatment for depression may be as simple as prescribing tranquilizers or it may be serious enough to require hospitalization. In some cases the doctor will prescribe shock therapy, a very dramatic procedure that has been used for many years.

Before the chemical revolution in psychiatry, shock therapy was often the best tool the psychiatrist had to treat depression. It took a great deal of dedication on the part of the doctor and a certain desperation on the part of the patient to make use of this procedure. It is still not understood how shock therapy works, and there is an ongoing disagreement as to whether it does work.

The therapy consists of a deliberate shock to the brain and nervous system by means of an insulin injection or an electrical charge. The shock seems to interrupt and restart the patient's brain activity, beginning a new period in the patient's life hopefully without the depression. The problem with the convulsive nature of shock therapy is that it causes a memory loss, sometimes short-term, sometimes permanent, and in some cases alters the patient's personality. It is no wonder that patients with depression and their doctors as well are pleased with the arsenal of medicines currently available.

Emotional Responses to P/D

Mental challenges are important to the P/D patient and to the caregiver alike in the maintenance of the give and take one finds in a marriage of some duration. Most mature adults have long established preferences in hobbies and recreational activities and it is wise to try to continue these or alternative activities when living with P/D.

In general, among those forced into retirement or inactivity by Parkinson's disease, there are several types of individuals represented.

First, there is the traditionalist. This is the dedicated hobbyist who couldn't wait for retirement so that he would have more time for his hobbies. He is the person who will continue old activities without interruption.

Second, there is the adventurer. This is the individual with the short attention span, who will try anything once and who sees a hundred things he wants to do. He, also, will not have a problem keeping himself amused.

The individual who has the most problems filling his days with activities is the third type, the workaholic who always intended to take up a hobby but was too busy with his work. He has never fished, played golf, watched birds, done woodworking or painted. This is the patient who can let himself develop an emotional problem if he is not helped and encouraged to get busy.

More Serious Problems

Continuing on the darker side of Parkinson's disease, unpleasant though it may seem, we recognize that in some instances of P/D mental problems are serious. These include night horrors, hallucinations, hostility, withdrawal, and when very advanced and untreated, dementia. These are not the most frequent problems encountered by Parkinsonians and they are beyond the scope of this book.

Both the Parkinsonian and the caregiver should realize that such extremes are not general; professional help and a variety of effective medicines are available. Relief is both possible and probable.

Psychological Coping 9

When a person is actively engaged in a program of physical conditioning quite often he will announce his intentions by wearing the colorful regalia of an athlete, a runner or whatever, sweats as they are casually called. He announces to the public that he is, or intends to be, physically fit. Unfortunately, there are no sweats to mark someone who may be working just as hard to attain a good state of mental health. This is especially hard for the Parkinson's disease patient who is struggling to keep a healthy mental attitude and whose success, or failure, may never be noticed, even by a loving spouse or a medical professional.

Recognizing And Coping With Change

Quite often psychological and emotional problems relating to P/D are difficult to evaluate or even to recognize. As a result, the patient often finds himself adrift on a sea of his own uncertainty, with a head full of thoughts, concerns, fears and unanswered questions, with no one, at least in his mind, to turn to for guidance or even understanding. Fortunately, the Parkinsonian has time to come to recognize the changes brought on by the disease, and to find his own way of coping with them.

He may be able to develop the needed insight on his own but, as is often the case, he will not accept the realities of his disease without drawing on the strengths and emotional stability of a spouse, a valued friend or a trusted professional. There are, undoubtedly, many P/D patients who feel comfortable with their clergyman and can benefit by his counsel, in which case I see no reason not to consult with him. My own feeling, however, is that the P/D patient is already under a lot of stress emotionally and does not need the guilt and the mysticism clerical counseling too often entails. Whomever the confidant, whatever his credentials, the one thing he needs to be is a good listener. I am convinced that a remarkably large portion of the emotional problems developed by P/D patients can be either alleviated or eliminated merely by vocalizing them, especially if they are heard by a caring listener.

No Vast Void

A newly diagnosed P/D patient is told that he has lost part of his brain cells, an important part to be sure, but he is almost never enlightened further on this score. So, the patient is left walking around with an image of himself as having a vast void in his head where his brain ought to be. A chilling, disabling thought and, of course, not true.

The precise number of brain cells actually lost is minute and there is no void as one might imagine it. The cells haven't gone anywhere, they have just quit making dopamine. I prefer to focus on the portions of the brain which remain alive and well, still capable of out-performing the most intelligent computer. Not only is the P/D patient left with most of his brain intact, he has the mental ability to find ways (sometimes with help, to be sure) to counteract and to compensate for the mobility and dexterity he has lost to P/D.

Avoiding Depression

As has already been said, depression is not the same thing as being depressed. Depression is an illness which can sap the energy of a patient and, if left untreated, can immobilize an otherwise healthy body. Depression is not something the patient can just talk his way out of. He needs help and that may mean professional counseling, chemical treatment by means of prescribed medication, or only the time of a caring, listening and available confidant. The patient in depression very likely knows in gross terms how or why he got into his depression. What he can't do is work out of it alone.

There has been a veritable revolution in the medicines available to treat depression. With the assortment of available drugs, there is a good prospect that the physician can prescribe medication which is effective, relatively free from side effects and comparatively inexpensive. It should be remembered and emphasized that living with depression is not really living.

The Parkinsonian has been deprived of his status as a wage earner. His role as a husband and a father has been altered and it is difficult to fulfill his image as a sportsman and as "just one of the boys." His sense of self-worth has hit rock bottom. Now, with help, the only direction he can go is up.

I keep coming back to the analogy of the mind being like a muscle, to use or to lose. For the Parkinsonian, it is still a good way to think as he strives for emotional fitness. The patient who is active mentally is less likely to become depressed and will be more capable of working his way out of a depression should it occur. So, how does one keep active mentally when the body seems determined to thwart every effort? I didn't say it was easy. But, it can be done.

To avoid depression or to reduce its impact and to aid in his own recovery, the P/D patient should seek out his confidant and verbalize his concerns. Talk about those fears: the fear of dying; the fear of not dying and becoming a burden to loved ones; the loss of self esteem; and, the feeling of isolation when family members and professionals discuss his condition in his presence as though he was no longer present.

In addition to vocalizing his problems, the P/D patient needs to work actively to exercise his mental muscle. Just as the patient has had to give up certain physical activities due to his disease he must give up, or modify, some mental activities. The emotional security provided by these activities must be compensated for through some other activity.

The possibilities are endless and limited only by the imagination of the patient, his interests of the past and his unfulfilled ambitions. In my own case, I retired early, at age 61, by my own decision, because I no longer enjoyed or felt fully competent in my work. I was in a field where most of my competitors and co-workers were half my age and possessed the stamina and enthusiasm to work long hours and to travel incessantly.

Since retiring, I have pursued previously unfulfilled interests in music, languages, calligraphy, celestial navigation, computer programming and have worked seriously as an aspiring writer. I am as busy now as I was when I was working. The difference is the absence of stress and comfort of a flexible routine.

If all the patient's best efforts fail to deal adequately with his depression then he should discuss with his physician the arsenal of drugs available.

Sleep Disturbances

Probably the next most frequent group of emotional problems among Parkinsonians is sleep disturbances, variously called nightmares, night horrors or by the medical term, Pavor Nocturnus. These are dreams which cause vocalization, agitation and violent movements which awaken the patient and spouse, and often make further sleep impossible. Other manifestations of these dreams are bruxism (grinding the teeth and clenching the jaws) and quite often cramps, especially of the leg.

These dreams defy analysis but almost certainly represent unresolved emotional conflicts which may, or may not, be related to Parkinson's disease. Since these dreams are often physically violent and a danger to the patient, as well as others, the physician will usually prescribe a mild sedative or sleeping pill to be taken at bedtime. This is not completely effective but it allows a more restful night of sleep.

Hallucinations

One of the most unsettling experiences for the P/D patient, and for those around him, is the initial and early onset of hallucinations and delusions which sometimes occur with some of the most effective medications for use in the treatment of symptoms of Parkinson's disease. Many physicians prescribe these powerful neuro-transmitters and neglect to give the patient and caregiver proper warning about hallucinations as a possible side effect. This sometimes leaves the patient and his spouse wondering if he is becoming a mental case when he sees figures, objects and people who seem to be there but aren't. This is not the case.

Although hallucinations are most often visual, (sometimes the figures seem distinct, three dimensional and almost recognizable) other examples may be nothing more than a draft of cold air where no draft should be, or an uncomfortable feeling of an undefinable presence on the back of one's chair or on the edge of the bed. The important thing is to remember that this is a common occurrence and should not be endured alone. The hallucinations are real but almost without exception they are drug-induced and can be satisfactorily explained by the physician in a few minutes.

When you do take the problem of hallucinations to your doctor be prepared to describe in some detail the nature of the hallucinations. The newspaper man's five "W"'s -- Who, What, When, Where and Why -- are a good way to examine what has been happening to the patient.

Negative Attitudes and Misinformation

In the struggle of the patient and his caregiver to maintain a healthy mental attitude as well as a healthy body, Juvenal said it quite well in his sixth satire in the second century AD: Mens Sana In Corpore Sano (Source uncertain). It is a good thing to review occasionally a list of persons whom the patient and the caregiver see frequently.

Almost any such list will have a name or two of persons who may be the salt of the earth in many ways yet will have a negative attitude sufficient to cause a depressed state of mind in the healthiest patient and caregiver. You owe it to yourself to put some distance between you and the negative personalities before they can inflict permanent damage.

The Parkinsonian can't go for very long without having someone, usually a non-professional with a head full of misinformation, linking Parkinson's disease and Alzheimers disease. While it is true that both are neuro-degenerative diseases the two should not be confused, linked or compared. The Parkinsonian and the Alzheimer's patient already have enough problems without compounding them.

One facet of Parkinson's disease one hears too much about is dementia. This severe impairment of intellectual capabilities, or cognition, is of interest to the Parkinsonian as a phenomenon in very advanced P/D, in extremis, and should not be a matter of great concern to the functioning Parkinsonian.

It is well, however, for the Parkinsonian and the caregiver to be aware of the fact that Parkinson's disease is not an entirely exclusive disease. Parkinsonians can and do have other diseases not related to P/D. While the medical community is not in as much of a hurry as they once were to label as senility any mental problems of the age group which includes most Parkinsonians, there is often a tendency to take short-sighted views of problems of the aging.

A Mental Checklist

To help the physician evaluate and identify problems of a mental and emotional nature and to screen for senility, the patient and the caregiver should ask themselves the following questions:

Is the patient's strange or erratic behavior random or does it follow a pattern?
Is the unusual behavior a gradually worsening problem, or did it start abruptly?
Is the patient aware of his behavior and is he able to logically explain his acts?

Is the patient able to control his eccentric behavior?
Is the patient's behavior a danger to himself or to others?
Has there been a physical or emotional trauma in the patient's life recently presenting more than usual stress?

Answering and discussing these questions will often explain behavioral problems without involving the physician, an example of self-help which can improve the state of mind of both the patient and the caregiver.

Physiological Effects 10

Although the usual view of Parkinson's disease is that it is primarily a physiological ailment with only peripheral psychological overtones, I had to make my own judgment on this. I believe that we are far more able to give up mobility and dexterity than we are the mental processes which shape our thoughts and words, giving breadth and depth to our personality. Who we are is not determined by our mobility or lack of it, but by the dimensions our minds can encompass. I have, therefore, given precedence to psychology over physiology in arranging the chapters of this book.

That is not to say that I take physical disabilities lightly. I do not.

It is a very frustrating thing to find one's ability to drive a car or fly a plane, to hop, skip or jump, to dance for joy, even to dress one's self or to turn over in bed to be diminished greatly or lost completely. The halting gait, feet shuffling and sliding unsteadily, the palsied hands and the weak voice seem to tell the world that here is a person who is less than whole. One cannot accept that status gracefully, one should not be expected to do so.

Overcoming Physical Difficulties

The disabilities cannot be denied but they can be contested, compensated for and confounded. If one keeps faith in himself and continues to be willing to fight, the physical aspects of Parkinson's disease can be made tolerable. With the time allowed us by the slow, if relentless, progress of the disease we have time to plan for disabilities to come.

While walking well unassisted is the time to be thinking of a cane. When using a cane one should consider a walker, and eventually a wheelchair. One should consider the progression from the conventional bed to one with handgrips and other assists to a hospital-type bed with rails and designed with mechanical features that allow the patient more mobility. Anything that makes it easier for the patient to sit up, turn over, and to get in and out of bed with less strain, should be things for the Parkinsonian family to anticipate and plan for.

The Threat of Falls

Though P/D is not life threatening it carries the potential of serious injury, especially from falls. A poll of any large group of Parkinsonians will reveal that more than half will admit to falling on a fairly frequent basis. Falling usually does not begin to be a problem until P/D is well advanced, though some patients begin to fall before the disease is diagnosed.

Falls are caused by a number of circumstances, among them the loss of pedal dexterity causing the patient to get his feet tangled in throw rugs, shag carpeting, raised door sills, and quite often in climbing stairs. Then, too, the Parkinsonian is likely to be troubled by festination, where the body gets ahead of the feet which take progressively shorter steps at a rapidly increasing rate until the patient falls. In these types of falls the tendency is to fall forward, resulting in some uncomfortable injuries.

Parkinsonians are prone to another type of fall which is the result of lowered blood pressure in the brain called Postural Hypotension. Postural Hypotension, a side effect of some medications used in treating the symptoms of P/D, can cause the patient to faint or "gray-out" when he gets up too abruptly from bed or a seated position. Unless this tendency is recognized and compensated for the patient is likely to fall or reel unsteadily until his blood pressure stabilizes (Sandoz Pharmaceuticals, 1989).

There is very little that the physician can do to help the patient avoid his tendency to fall. The patient and the caregiver, however, can institute a study of the falls to determine when and how the patient falls and make a plan to reduce the hazards, frequency and severity of his falls.

It is very important that the patient be protected from falls, but not at all costs. If the patient is sheltered and protected too much he may be prevented from engaging in some of his most rewarding activities. In my case, I still ride my bicycle though I know that I am likely to take an occasional fall. The rewards are a feeling of accomplishment plus a very good workout. I protect myself with a helmet, gloves, sturdy shoes and some strategic padding.

Most Parkinsonians will tell you that incidence of emotional stress is much more frequent when, for some reason, the daily exercise routine is interrupted. Physical injuries can cause a deterioration in the emotional health as well as the physical well-being of a patient. Once again the patient, the caregiver and the physician are caught up in a balancing act of the hazards of inactivity versus the protection of the patient from injury. It doesn't require the wisdom of

Solomon to realize that for the Parkinsonian the choice is clear. Maintaining the maximum fitness of body is imperative, repeating, once again the old maxim, "Use it or lose it." This brings us to yet another dilemma faced by Parkinsonians, the problem of fatigue.

Dealing With Fatigue

The weakening of muscle groups throughout the body and the loss of range of movements of skeletal joints as Parkinson's disease progresses leaves the patient stiff, weak and frustrated. The question of fatigue arises and the Parkinsonian must ask himself, "How much fatigue is too much?"

The aerobics instructor might say, "Work it till it hurts." The loving spouse might say, "You've done enough today. Take a rest." The doctor is likely to say, "The patient is the best judge. Exercise until you are physically challenged and emotionally calm." After much advice and discussion, the Parkinsonian is right where he was before. He is certain that he should do something but uncertain as to how much he should do. My solution is to set goals for myself or an agenda if you prefer.

I have found that muscle strength and joint flexibility achieved after a good workout persist for several days. Therefore, I work on a different group each day. One day I concentrate on the forearm and hand, another day on deep breathing and endurance. These routines need not be formal workouts. In fact, it is probably better if exercises can be integrated into one's daily routine, using a broomstick or two cans of tomatoes to strengthen those muscles.

There are countless possibilities around the home that can be pressed into service in an exercise and fitness program.

The idea that a fully equipped home gymnasium is necessary is a merchandising ploy, nothing more. In fact, just the exertion of getting out of bed or rising from a chair, if properly done and repeated frequently, can be physically challenging.

The Absence of Pain

One physical aspect of Parkinson's disease that I haven't mentioned in the foregoing discussions is the matter of pain, or perhaps I should say, absence of pain. Despite the many problems of P/D, the indignities and inconveniences heaped on the Parkinsonian, physical pain is not a factor. The Parkinsonian loses mobility and joint flexibility but the only pain he suffers is in his wallet.

Though pain is rarely, if ever, associated with P/D just about every aspect of daily living is apt to be a physical and an emotional challenge, something to be fought against with weapons we already have in our possession, grit and perspicacity. What has been said before on many occasions bears repeating:

> *"Illegitimus Non Carborundum!" Don't let the blankedy- blank disease wear you down! (Source uncertain.)*

Physiological Coping 11

Physiological coping, or the need for it, is with the Parkinsonian from the minute he wakes up in the morning until he falls asleep at night. It often intrudes during the night, preventing restful sleep. For purposes of this discussion let's start when the patient awakens in the morning.

A Typical Scenario

The Parkinsonian awakens to the same stimuli as the man down the street. The sun comes up, an alarm goes off, street noises intrude, the habits of a long working life provide a jab to the senses at some apparently preordained time. But while the man down the street awakens, yawns, scratches his head, throws back the covers, sits up in bed, puts his feet on the floor, puts on a robe and slippers and heads for the bathroom in a coordinated set of motions so automatic and so casual as to be accomplished without a thought, this is not the case for the Parkinsonian.

Getting Out of Bed

The Parkinsonian, his body and his brain deprived of medication through a long night, most often awakens to tremors of the hands, arms, legs, and the whole body. He must think of how to get the covers thrown back. Most often, all he can do is to push them aside. To sit up in bed is next to impossible.

If the patient is sufficiently strong and mobile he can roll onto his side, put one, or both, legs over the side while pushing his torso upright with both arms to sit on the edge of the bed. He sits there for a full minute or more for two reasons. First, some P/D medicines cause lowered blood pressure and abrupt changes of position can cause a feeling of fainting, dizziness or blackouts. Second, it is not easy for the Parkinsonian to get up from a seated position and it may take several bounces on the edge of the bed for him to get to a standing position. Again, it is important to have something to hold on to while the blood pressure stabilizes.

Then, the struggle with the robe. Fingers, hands and arms have all lost dexterity and strength. You no longer have the ability to put on a robe easily. Each Parkinsonian must find his own way to cope. For some a slip-over garment is easier to get into. Others use kimono-type robes with wide sleeves.

Slippers are also a problem. Most scuffs, mules and sandals do not provide sure footing and preferably should not be used. Moccasin or loafer shoes are better, preferably with a leather or composition sole, not slippery yet not sticky like crepe soles. A long-handled shoe horn, kept in sight and near at hand, is almost a necessity.

It is vital that the Parkinson's disease patient have a fixed place for all the necessities required by an aging person, Parkinsonian or not. Glasses, teeth, hearing-aid, watch, handkerchief and cane, to name a few, all should have a definite location, safe but accessible.

Now, back to our story.

The Parkinson is already 15 minutes into his day and has just now made it to the bathroom, while the man down the street has finished his morning ablutions and is sitting down to breakfast.

Bathroom Necessities

The Parkinsonian needs unhurried time in the bathroom. Sitting on and rising from the toilet may require the installation of handgrips to help steady the patient. Often it may be preferable for the patient to wait until the "turn-on" of his morning medicine to shave, brush his teeth or comb his hair. The bath or shower definitely should wait until after "turn-on".

In the bathroom, the Parkinsonian needs all the help he can get. An electric razor, electric toothbrush, large handles for hair and bath brushes, a shower head on a hose, a seat for the bathtub and one to use in front of the lavatory, all can be helpful. So can soap on a rope and the push-pump dispensers for tooth paste, shaving cream, and shampoo.

Reminding the druggist to leave off the childproof caps on medicine bottles is a simple coping ploy that far too many Parkinsonians neglect to use for themselves. A washcloth mitt is handy for the bath, and toweling off while seated eliminates concern over falling.

Don't forget the medicine. Take it first thing. To help eliminate the struggle with the bottles, ask the druggist for straight-sided containers instead of bottles with small necks. Be careful not to drop a $150.00 bottle of Parlodel in the toilet. Remember to take pills and capsules singly, and take care to coordinate breathing and swallowing so as not to get choked.

Finished with the bathroom for the time being. Lapsed time: 20 to 30 minutes.

Morning Routine

Now, head for the kitchen for some breakfast. On the way look at the barometer and at the morning sky to determine what the day's activity might be. Turn on the television and rewind the VCR with last night's Johnny Carson show. And, now, breakfast.

Wherever one has breakfast it should be convenient, safe and pleasant. I usually eat breakfast at a bar in the kitchen, sitting on a stool where I can see the television. I watch a few minutes of news, weather and business switching channels like mad.

The remote controls for TV and VCR are a great convenience and we use them for all our sets.

My breakfast varies from season to season and changes as I grow tired of one thing or another. Usually, I have melon or grapefruit, or juice, a scrambled egg or egg substitute, two slices of bacon or link sausage or their substitutes, a slice of all grain toast with margarine and black coffee in a mug with a generous, easy-to-grasp handle. Large-handled eating utensils are available if the patient feels more comfortable with them. As to napkins, I use a generous-sized cloth napkin which stays on the knees better. Eat and drink slowly, (as if a Parkinsonian could eat fast!) taking care not to get choked. I take my second mug of coffee to my easy chair in the family room to watch the Carson show, waiting for the medicine to "turn on" and planning the day's activities.

Most physicians have their P/D patients leave off their medication overnight, saving the precious benefits of dopamine for waking hours. The wait of 30 minutes to an hour before the effects of the medicine are felt can be frustrating if you let it. I devote this interim to planning my activity for the day. Some days you "turn on" better than others so your planned activity must be flexible. Following is a typical "good" day for me:

> *Up at 5:30, no particular reason, (some days earlier, some days later). Through with breakfast and Johnny Carson by 7:00. To the computer to check the overnight markets, at the word processor to write a letter about a high school reunion.*
>
> *The weather is nice so I dress to work outside. Heavy work this morning, building a patio of paving blocks set in sand. Dress in bedroom where spouse has clothes on hooks behind door, easy access. Suspenders instead of a belt, velcro closures on shoes. Slow process on dressing. Underwear, shirt, pants, socks and shoes take 15 minutes. Spend five minutes with a pair of 3 kg dumbbells (about 7 pounds) to loosen up arm and shoulder muscles.*
>
> *Work outside four hours, shoveling earth, wheelbarrow hauling, placing sand, leveling sand and placing 20 pound locks. Medicine at 11:00. Lunch outdoors on a tray. Read mail, admire morning's work, recreational reading, check stockticker until medicine turns on. Afternoon at word processor on newspaper column. Talk with broker using phone amplifier. Afternoon nap, one hour. Check market close on ticker. Medication at 4:00,*

> *light dinner. Four light meals instead of three ordinary meals. Afterward, spend one or two hours writing on current project(s).*
>
> *Compare notes with spouse on day's activities and plan tomorrow's activity, subject to weather. After catching up on local and world news, outside to look at flowers, check birdbath, water plants. Then, back to the computer to fly the flight simulator or play chess for an hour, sometimes shorter games. A sandwich and a glass of milk, then settle down for a couple of hours of TV, something on A & E, Bravo, Discovery or PBS. Some network programs, "Night Court", "The Cosby Show", "L.A. Law" and a few others. I usually change to PJs, a robe and slippers early in the evening, depending on how I feel and what kind of work I have been doing.*

The physical exertion part of the day can vary. It may be a 10-mile bike ride, five miles in my kayak or a brisk three-mile walk to pick up a newspaper. (Don't let them deliver your papers. It makes you lazy.) Not every Parkinson's disease patient can do this much. Some can do less, others can do more. It is a choice each patient must make for himself.

Bedtime Routine

Bedtime for me is 11:00 p.m. Getting ready for bed is a slow process. A final trip to the bathroom. Brush teeth, put glasses, hearing aid, watch in their overnight spot, and place pillows and bedding just so or the night will not go well. Take a quick check of the several nightlights scattered over the house.

I look at the smoke detectors and door locks and make a final check of the VCR programming before taking a sleeping pill and going to bed. An electric clock, digital with two-inch numerals, keeps me on track as far as the passing of the night is concerned. Sleeping arrangements and accouterments can be a source of great discomfort or great satisfaction dependent upon whether one has taken his affliction with P/D into consideration or persists in trying to continue with old habits held over from earlier times.

Tips for a More Restful Night

First and foremost, the Parkinsonian should arrange to sleep alone. Getting through the night while trying to sleep with a Parkinsonian can be equated with cruel and unusual punishment. We are discussing sleeping together. There is no reason to give up waking hours in bed together for sex or companionship but, for the well being of both partners, do your sleeping alone.

Sheets, Pillows, etc.

In the earlier stages of P/D there are usually no special arrangements required for sleeping other than a firm, comfortable mattress and a bedframe with casters that lock or have been removed so that the bed does not move when the patient is getting in or out of bed. Having tried a lot of variations in bedding we have settled on cotton sheets and pillow cases.

Many patients swear by satin sheets because they are slippery and are supposed to make it easier to maneuver in bed. The assistance I received from satin sheets was minimal and not worth the expense and the added effort required in making the bed and keeping it made.

I like down pillows but as an allergy sufferer the synthetic fillers are my choice, although I believe quality down is satisfactory for most people. I keep two pillows, one plump, one flat. I combine or alternate these, depending upon whether my stiff neck is bothering me.

In summertime, a sheet and a light thermal blanket are sufficient cover for me. In winter, I add a light electric blanket and this is all I need in the moderate climate we enjoy in east Tennessee. I have tried down comforters but they are expensive, slippery and difficult to keep in place as well as their potential effect on allergies.

A bookcase headboard on the bed is a good thing to have for everyone, including Parkinsonians. It serves as a repository for eye drops, nose drops, throat lozenges, tissues, a note pad and a ballpoint pen, prism glasses for watching TV from a supine position, the TV and VCR remote controls, a telephone and a small telephone amplifier.

I have two incandescent light fixtures securely fastened to the headboard and controlled with a dimmer. The headboard holds my current reading matter plus old standbys and references, World Almanac, dictionary, an atlas, Bartlett's quotations, collected works of Thoreau, Conan Doyle, Shakespeare, Mark Twain and Opera Scores and Librettos. A flashlight and a weather radio complete the inventory except for two items I want to discuss a bit.

Two 'Special' Items

The first of these is a dark, padded, satin sleep mask with an elastic headband. I use it for a problem not unique with me. I sleep in a prone position much of the time and I drool on my pillow or the sheet in copious amounts. During the night I get saliva in my eyes causing uncomfortable and unsightly irritation. The mask eliminates that problem.

The other item may be of interest to others and not just Parkinsonians. It is an inexpensive biofeedback device that I use to help me control the pain of migraine headaches. I have always been headache prone and have tried all the various forms of treatment including Caefergot which made me sicker than the migraine. I have no reason to believe that the headaches are related to Parkinson's disease in any way since they predate the P/D by more than 50 years.

The biofeedback device is simply a compact electronic device which generates an audible signal which, when biased by the input of electrodes connected to two fingers of one hand, changes tone according to the level of electric energy in the brain. This energy level, monitored by a small earphone can be controlled by a learned conscious technique and reduced to a level which, when properly done, masks the pain of a headache until the patient is able to go to sleep, that being the best relief. I have found that an ice-bag applied to the solar plexus during and after biofeedback therapy contributes to the relief of headache symptoms.

Sleepware

For the Parkinsonian there is no ideal nightwear and many patients, not having been able to find suitable garments, have elected to sleep in the nude. I am not comfortable sleeping nude and I have, after trying a variety of pajamas, (long, short, soft and slippery) settled on cotton knit nightshirts as being the least binding and the easiest for getting in and out of bed.

To bed at last, after a long day. The Parkinsonian is once more just like the man down the street until the Parkinsonian awakens from a nightmare or a need to urinate. Getting up at night can be risky but can be made safer with the use of nightlights and by removing hazards. A walker kept handy can reduce hazards for that trip to the bathroom and you eventually will want to consider keeping a urinal at bedside for safety and convenience.

Things No One Will Talk About 12

Most Parkinsonians are persons in the age group 50 and older. They grew up in a time when they were inhibited or constrained about openly discussing certain subjects in interviews with medical professionals, in support groups or even with a spouse of many years.

It seems somehow incongruous that mature adults with a need to know often go uninformed about some of the effects that Parkinson's disease has on the patient and his spouse, specifically sexual and excretory problems. In addition to the patient's reluctance to broach these problems with his doctor there is the all too frequent circumstance that the physician, especially if he is also in the Parkinsonian age group, may not be prepared to knowledgeably discuss sexual concerns and incontinence.

The Parkinsonian and his caregiver are urged to overcome their reticence in these areas and to find a physician who is comfortable and knowledgeable with the problems of sexual dysfunction. Since P/D involves almost every facet of one's life, concerns about sexual problems should not be allowed to go unasked and unresolved.

Sexual Concerns

A discussion of Parkinson's disease and the problems it can cause the patient in the expression of sex drive is made more difficult by the almost universal reticence of persons in the P/D age group to talk frankly with their spouse or a professional who might conceivably be able to help. This is unfortunate because an understanding spouse and open exchange of ideas and opinions can make sex an enriching and rewarding part of the lives of both the patient and spouse, despite changes brought about by advancing age and the progress of the disease.

This lack of communication existed before the advent of P/D and generally is reinforced by the psychological problems engendered by the disease. This makes the problem of dealing with changes in one's sex life especially difficult. The Parkinsonian's problems with sex are not so much physical as they are emotional, much like other adjustments the P/D couple must make. Therefore, this discussion will not be as much a "how to" guide as it will be an examination of ways and means to elicit an open and honest expression of the needs of both partners. As is the case in so many other examples of coping behavior the realities of Parkinson's disease are that changes of lifestyle are almost always necessary. These changes should not be bemoaned. Rather, they should be regarded as an opportunity for insight and growth.

Adjustments in Sexual Expression

With the advance of P/D symptoms, the sexual techniques, habits and preferences of half a lifetime may have to be discarded or drastically altered. The former instigator or innovator may now become a seemingly passive or disinterested participant. Care must be taken to go beyond mere superficial appearances and look at the reasons for the apparent disinterest and non- participation. Though adjustments may need to be made in one's sex life, it is worthwhile.

Adjustments in the expression of sexual needs must, of necessity, vary widely because manifestations of the disease are as varied as those in the other categories. Foreplay may become more or less important than before and autoerotism may become a part of the sexual expression of the Parkinsonian couple, whether or not it was used previously. New or revised autoerotic techniques may fill a need for the couple, together or individually, to compensate for absent or reduced capabilities of the partner.

Typical Sexual Problems

Problems of a sexual nature that are most prevalent vary from difficulty in getting and maintaining an erection; slowed, erratic or missing ability to perform the tempo and vigor of the necessary thrusting motions; premature or delayed ejaculation; and, loss of ability to achieve orgasm. Regardless of how P/D affects a man in other ways, sexual expression or damages to his performance in a sexual way can strike a calamitous blow to the male self-image if not treated with care and respect.

The sexual problems of women Parkinsonians can and do vary as widely as among men. The more frequent problems are loss of vaginal lubrication; involuntary loss of urine during intimacy; stiffness of joints; disconcerting cramps or tremors at inappropriate times; and, loss of movement and rhythm.

In the early stages of P/D the patient and spouse may not be aware of diminishing sexual capabilities, but as time passes both partners are affected and suffer the loss. Teamwork and honest expression of one's needs and preferences should be used as a tool to deal with the problems.

The Search for New Techniques

Outside of sharing more readily the information on needs, preferences and problems, the next most desirable area for discussion and change may be the search for fresh or different techniques. These may consist of variations of foreplay habits, changes in the time and place in which one engages in sexual activity, and the use of marital aids.

Serious consideration of the practice of autoerotism, or masturbation, through reading and discussing the custom together or with an enlightened professional counselor will make it clear that autoerotism is an acceptable sexual outlet. It should not be considered as a betrayal of the partner whether it is practiced together or alone in the privacy of the bedroom or bath when sexual needs require a release.

An investment in one or more of the many guides or manuals on a more varied sex life can bring rewards far beyond their cost for the Parkinsonian couple struggling to prevent the loss of one of life's most basic drives.

Pornography, in soft- or hard-core varieties, is reasonably priced and is widely available in printed form and on video cassettes. For the Parkinsonian couple and especially the P/D patient living alone, this small amount of tittilation may be just what is needed to overcome the inertia which prevents many Parkinsonian's and their spouses from maintaining any kind of sexual involvement. Sex manuals, pornographic magazines and explicit sex on video cassettes are, of course, subject to individual preferences. However, it is my feeling that one should not discard options of the present on the basis of moral judgments of a half-century ago.

An interesting aside to the subject of the sex lives of Parkinsonians relates to the early days of L-Dopa therapy. There was a lot of snickering and ribald comment when the media and the general public became aware that one of the more uncommon side effects of L-Dopa was that it caused priapism or clitorism in some patients. These erections, though they were genuine, had nothing to do with libido. They did nothing toward providing an erotic plus to the sex life of the Parkinsonian and most often came to be regarded as an uncomfortable nuisance. (So much for folk lore.)

A good thought for the P/D couple to remember: "A great sex life begins in the brain, not the genitalia."

Professional Counsel

Beyond the self-help aspects of sexual activity for the Parkinsonian there is always the option of seeking the counsel of a medical professional. The difficulty with this course of action is in finding a practitioner who is qualified and competent, and the process may lead to disappointment.

Medical schools do not seem to provide the knowledge and insight to their students which will enable them to successfully counsel patients with the sexual dysfunction which occurs with Parkinson's disease. There are some individuals in the medical profession who are effective counselors, most frequently, (so it seems to me) on the basis of an innate sensitivity rather than through some course of study. The effort required to find this individual can be worthwhile for the Parkinsonian and should be pursued if one is not satisfied with this important aspect of his life.

Dealing With Incontinence

Since Parkinson's disease affects motor or muscle functions throughout the body it should not be too difficult to see that excretory problems are the result of malfunctions of the various sphincter muscles which control the voiding of urine and feces. Though it is not specifically excretory, the pyloric sphincter in the digestive tract can be considered in the same context.

Urinary Problems

The first manifestation of urinary problems for the Parkinsonian is a sudden urge to urinate which is independent of volume of the bladder contents or of recent liquid intake. Frequently, this urge will be overpowering for a short time and will then subside without voiding any urine.

This may recur several times and when the patient does urinate the volume and the force of the stream may vary widely, seemingly unrelated to the amount of discomfort one has suffered. As Parkinson's disease progresses these urges to urinate are often accompanied by spasm-like relaxations of the bladder sphincter with the involuntary discharge of urine, a few drops, a few spurts, or the entire contents of the bladder.

The loss of urine amounts to 1 to 4 ounces or more (25 ml to 125 ml or more) in a paroxysm which can be uncomfortable, embarrassing and inconvenient. In theory, at least, this loss of urine at inconvenient times could or should be controlled by reducing the intake of fluids prior to an inconvenient time period. However, this doesn't always work.

In male Parkinsonians, especially, it is important that the patient be seen by a urologist to rule out problems of the urinary tract such as an enlarged prostate or anything requiring medication.

Assuming that the urologist has satisfied himself and the patient that there is no other problem, the Parkinsonian can set about living with this problem which seems much more embarrassing to the patient than it is to others. The purchase and use of absorbent sleeves, pads or undergarments, now widely available, reduces some of the uncertainty in the mind of the Parkinsonian and allows him to resume a more nearly normal routine.

Probably the best strategy for dealing with bladder incontinence is to take steps to control the embarrassment and concern and to avoid, as much as possible, complicating P/D treatment with medicine for urinary problems.

At night one of the worst hazards of those nocturnal visits to the bathroom is the danger of falling for this is when the Parkinsonian is most vulnerable. If the hazards become too great it may be a good idea to keep a urinal by the bedside, making those nightly trips unnecessary.

Digestive Disorders

The first problem the Parkinsonian notices with his digestive system is an increase of flatulence, an increase of intestinal gas, which is not peculiar to Parkinsonians but is a problem shared by many in the P/D age group. As the ability to control the anal sphincter is lost it becomes more and more difficult to distinguish between the voiding of a flatus, a bubble of gas, and involuntary excretion of feces. For the fastidious adult this loss of control is a source of embarrassment and shame, and that is the principal problem that needs to be solved.

Assuming that there are no complications in the digestive tract -- something which should be discussed with the primary physician -- the patient needs to work on overcoming his embarrassment at becoming incontinent. This leaves only the actual control of the products of that incontinence, which is as simple as purchasing and using suitable absorbent undergarments and exercising more care in maintaining the best possible state of health for regulation of bowel movements.

The principal complaint of Parkinsonians as to elimination is that of constipation. All too often the P/D patient relies on self-help and over-the-counter remedies to regulate his bowel habits. This impatience and misunderstanding of elimination can lead to a worsening of the problem instead of improvement. The Parkinsonian with a problem of irregularity should consult with his physician.

Rest assured, however, accidents will happen at the most inconvenient and embarrassing times. I choose to think of the perpetrator of these acts of incontinence on the Parkinsonian as being a doppleganger, a double or shadow with a sense of time and a mind of his own, out to embarrass the Parkinsonian.

The necessity for wearing absorbent undergarments is a small inconvenience to avoid the feeling of being a pariah.

Helpful Hints 13

Perambulation

The heretofore simple task of getting about becomes increasingly complicated for the Parkinsonian. In the early stages of the disease it may amount to a slight tremor of the hand as you attempt to put a key in a lock or, as you try to negotiate a tricky set of steps, your toe drops inexplicably and you fall sprawling. As the disease progresses so do the problems of getting about. The patient finds that he must compensate in strange ways for his loss of mobility.

One of the first ploys the Parkinsonian learns is the "bounce" used to get from a sitting position to a standing position. This maneuver uses the resilience of springs in a bed or chair to assist you in rising. Two or three bounces with increasing intensity will often compensate for loss of muscular strength and joint stiffness.

Controlling Inertia

In the home, the Parkinsonian has a tendency to shuffle rather than to stride. This is a natural compensation for loss of motor function. It should be fought as long as one can do it safely.

Striding is preferable but fast, positive movements, once initiated, generate inertia which then makes it difficult to stop or even to turn. The initiation of a movement (or the termination of one) is further complicated by variations in motor function capabilities brought on by the "on and off" cycle of the medication. In the "off" periods, the Parkinsonian will begin festination, a walking pattern in which he takes progressively shorter steps at a rapidly increasing rate until he is walking furiously in place or becomes unbalanced and falls.

The P/D patient may find that he needs to divide a trip from one room to another, say from the family room to the bathroom, into increments. For example:

> *"Bounce" out of the easy chair. "Steady" the upright posture by grasping the chair to make sure that rising has not made you faint, lightheaded or dizzy. "Lurch" to the door. "Grasp" the doorframe. "Stride" through the living room. "Push off" at the bathroom corner. Then, "veer" into the bathroom.*

This is what I call my controlled trajectory.

Out of doors the venue is less restrictive but no less hazardous. There is more striding and less shuffle, fewer push-offs and better veers. The problem of overcoming inertia out of doors is complex.

Though inertia cannot be done away with, it can be controlled. Carrying something weighty in one or both hands can salvage and enhance the natural rhythms of walking. What to carry is the patient's choice. It may be a cane, an umbrella or exercise weights strapped to wrists and ankles. After movement has been initiated and a reasonably natural pace has been established care must be taken to avoid tripping and slipping hazards. Be aware of vehicles and other pedestrians, and above all pace yourself so as not to go beyond endurance.

Climbing/Descending Steps

One of the most difficult things to ask of a Parkinsonian is to have him climb steps. Here, all the adverse effects of P/D come into play. The stiff joints, the loss of muscle tone, the effects of gravity, the toe drop on one or both feet, combine to trap and immobilize the Parkinsonian.

Descending steps can be just as hazardous. The tendency of Parkinsonians to lean forward is often just enough unbalance to cause a fall. A split-level or a tri-level house can be a trial for the P/D patient and a lot of consideration should be given to this problem soon after the disease is diagnosed. I knew I had P/D when we bought our retirement home and we had the luxury of looking for just the right house. Not everyone will be able to do as I did but the home and future immobility require some thought and planning.

Retaining Mobility

The previous discussion may give the impression that we are considering only the ambulatory P/D patient. The ambulatory stage of P/D lasts the longest, therefore the longer discussion. We are not ignoring the possibility, and the probability, that those with P/D usually go from unassisted walking to a cane, then to a walker and finally to a wheelchair. What we want to do is increase the length of time each stage can be perpetuated.

Sometimes, in a desire to protect the patient from falls and injury, the caregiver may be overprotective of the Parkinsonian to his detriment as far as mobility is concerned. Falls are bad and injuries do occur, but the patient needs to keep all the mobility he has for as long as he can. Even if this means putting him in a helmet with elbow and knee pads, this is preferable to having the patient so cloistered that he is afraid to move without assistance.

My own legs look like a disaster area from getting tangled in my bicycle pedals, but I still manage to ride seven to 10 healthful miles whenever I like. The same goes for my kayak. I don't swim as well as I once did so I do make a concession of always wearing a flotation device, even in calm waters where I can do five to eight miles with relative ease.

Even the adoption of a wheelchair need not put an end to pride in mobility for the patient. Plan together to have the patient, in his wheelchair, give the caregiver a break occasionally. It is not an imposition on the patient to have him help with the laundry, to prepare a snack or light meal and to wash up afterwards. It takes some planning but the pride of accomplishment for the patient and the satisfaction for the caregiver in keeping the patient involved is, and should be, considerable.

Manual Tasks

With the advance of his disease the patient finds his loss of dexterity to be substantial and disturbing. Without realizing it, he may begin to compensate for abilities he has lost. Keys get transferred to the opposite hand, a different hand is used to open doors, and wheel-holding styles change when the patient is driving an automobile. Lost motor skills can be compensated for by ingenuity and hard work.

Coping With Handwriting Loss

Fast and legible handwriting quickly disappears. The first compensations are to write less, to work at making it larger and to practice using block letter printing. A small cassette tape recorder can be a real life saver for taking notes.

I find, now, that I am more comfortable with a typewriter or computer keyboard than with a traditional pen or pencil. I have a small battery powered typewriter, a portable weighing about five pounds which I take everywhere with me. It is fast and quiet and unobtrusive.

At home I still use my old IBM electric typewriter, a Commodore computer with Geos software and a Brother word processor. I also use a tape recorder and a VCR to help me through the day.

Keep Hands Active

Despite the loss of function, care should be taken that the hands are not allowed to grow soft and weak from lack of use. If there is not enough physical activity in the patient's normal routine to keep his grip firm he should be encouraged to squeeze a tennis ball, alternating hands, several times a day, to use spring-type handgrips or light dumbbells. Any repetitious hand activity can provide therapy for unused fingers and hands. Shuffling and dealing cards, playing a piano, operating a loom, working at wood carving or on a potter's wheel, laying brick for a wall, and doing needle point, are only a few of the many options chosen by Parkinsonians. The list is limited only by the imagination of the patient.

It should not be lost to the patient that therapeutic exercise should be timed to coincide with the "ups" or "ons" of his medicine's cycle. Things he can do to perfection while "on" can be a disaster when he is "off". Observance of these cycles is essential to the patient's emotional well-being.

Eyesight

The sense of sight is a complex and delicately balanced process which is still not perfectly understood by medical professionals and which is far beyond the scope of this book to discuss in detail.

It must be recognized that eyesight is affected by Parkinson's disease in strange and diverse ways, complicated by the fact that the patient may have vision problems relating to the aging process or to eye diseases having nothing to do with P/D. It is essential to the full visual health of the Parkinsonian that the patient and caregiver discuss with a knowledgeable ophthalmologist changes in eyesight observed after the diagnosis of P/D has been confirmed. With something as valuable as one's sight, the P/D patient owes it to himself and to his family to schedule regular visits to the ophthalmologist.

Too Simple a Comparison

The comparison, often made, of the eye and a camera is much too simple a comparison. The vision apparatus has sensory and motor connections, tear and tear film functions and a complex arrangement of nerves. There is an optic nerve which exits the back of each eye, and which contains thousands of individual fibers. The two optic nerves meet at a nerve crossing (or chiasma) where about half of the nerve fibers cross to the opposite side of the chiasma and others do not. This discussion has to do with the left and right visual field, or the area covered by that part of the eye.

The visual field of each eye is divided into a nasal and a temporal half. The nasal fibers cross at the chiasma and go to the opposite side of the brain. All of the optic sensory nerves end up in the vision center in the occipital cerebral cortex at the posterior or back of the brain.

Vision Problems and P/D

It is obvious that the sense of sight is complex in the normal healthy individual and it is doubly so when complicated by Parkinson's disease. Attributing vision problems to P/D is a risky business since the aging process produces some of the same symptoms noticed by the Parkinsonian.

Among these symptoms are slow adjustment of the eyes to changing light levels, a reduction of the visual field, reduced range of movement of the eyes, dry eyes and impairment of binocular vision. Some forms of conjunctivitis, iritis and glaucoma found in the P/D age group probably have no direct connection to aging or to Parkinson's disease.

Once again, let me emphasize that this discussion is intended to stress the complexity of the visual sense and the need for the opinion of an ophthalmologist. I have found, by my own observations, that I have lost a substantial amount of night vision, a common complaint in the Parkinsonian age group. My motor function in moving my eyes rapidly (up and down or right and left) is impaired. My eyelid blink rate has dropped to practically zero, and my eyes are dry most of the time, requiring the use of artificial tears.

Another vision peculiarity I have noticed, is that at night before going to sleep or just after awakening, I sometimes experience a spasm-like flutter of the eyelids which makes the dim light of a nightlight seem to have a stroboscopic effect. It sometimes takes a touch or a rub of the eyelid to stop the flutter.

Another phenomenon I have noticed in the dark of night is a kind of double vision. I experience this only in looking at the illuminated large red numerals of a digital clock where I sometimes see two distinct images of the display, separated by an approximate distance of one display vertically and horizontally. The image for the left or dominant eye is the higher of the two. I attribute this to a strange type of suppression of the vision of the subordinate right eye by the dominant left eye, a condition which is not connected to my P/D.

I refer to these vision problems of mine not so much because I expect other Parkinsonians to have similar problems but to try to convey the needs and complexity of the sense of sight and admonition to see your ophthalmologist.

Swallowing, Breathing, Speech Difficulties

The Parkinson's disease patient has problems with swallowing, breathing and speech which are difficult if not impossible to separate. I have chosen to consider them as a group. These problems have a symbiotic relationship, develop slowly but insidiously. The best defense against these problems is an informed and aggressive offense.

Loss of lung capacity and of ribcage flexibility may go unnoticed for a long time because the condition takes so long to develop. Lack of exercise is all too common in persons during the early stages of P/D when the tendency is for the patient to give up on any physical activity which has some degree of difficulty. What he is remiss in considering is, that in order to maintain good cardiovascular health, it is necessary to increase by exercise the heart and respiration rates for 15 to 30 minutes four or five times a week. Respiration is a complex process which involves not only the flexibility of the chest wall but the diaphragm as well, the diaphragm being a membranous muscle.

I have found that the pulse rate is a better indicator of physical conditioning than respiration rate. Here is a formula that I have used for over 10 years to monitor my heart rate during exercise. It considers age as a component and it has worked well for me: 220-AGE X .80 = MAXIMUM HEART RATE.

Using this formula an otherwise healthy Parkinsonian at age 65 should be able to exercise to a heart rate of approximately 124. Exercise is important. Get your physician's advice and consent before you begin an exercise program. Begin slowly and increase as you feel the need.

Speech Difficulties

Speech difficulties with P/D arise from more than one cause. Loss of muscle tone in the jaw, lips and tongue, the throat and diaphragm, and dissimilarities between the muscles of the left and right sides can cause difficulty with enunciation, pronunciation, volume and projection. Fricative sounds which require thrusting the tongue forward toward or against the teeth become noticeably more difficult. The vocal cords, which form the components of speech, are also muscles which are affected by the loss of tone as well as variations in the "off/on" of the Parkinsonian's medication cycle.

Speech consists of many components but chiefly involves expulsion of air from the lungs through the larynx forming the basic sounds of one's voice. The formation of these sounds into recognizable speech involves the hard and soft palates and the lips and tongue, naming only the principal components.

Speech therapy is often not necessary for the Parkinsonian in the early or immediate stages of the disease. But, this is the time for the P/D patient to begin to make use of the expertise of the professional speech therapist to improve and to prolong the ability to speak so that others will understand. It is nearly impossible for the patient to be objective about the volume, tempo and clarity of his speech.

The patient is hindered in making his own evaluation because of sinus resonances and uncertainty of acoustics and sound levels. A speech therapist, however, will conduct a hearing evaluation at a number of frequencies using accurately calibrated equipment in scientifically designed acoustical surroundings. On the basis of these tests, the therapist can recommend speech exercises and drills designed to keep the vocal apparatus functioning as nearly normal as is possible with the Parkinson's disease. He will also counsel the patient on his speech strengths and weaknesses and will describe how to make use of one and compensate for the other, including advice on hearing loss and the present or future need for a hearing aid.

A useful tool for speech therapy exercises is a small cassette tape recorder with a legible VU or sound level meter and a sound activated microphone. A half hour of reciting or reading aloud three or four times a week can be beneficial, especially when practiced before a mirror. Taking care to project one's voice and to enunciate clearly has an added benefit in that these exercises get us out of our lazy speech patterns, a benefit to everyone, not just Parkinsonians. When the P/D patient no longer has good speech volume, electronic amplifiers are available.

Swallowing Dysfunctions

Swallowing is another complex function which, when examined in detail, seems next to impossible to perform properly, even by a normal healthy human being. It is no wonder then, with the dysfunction that he has to contend with, that the Parkinsonian has swallowing and choking problems.

Swallowing is almost always initiated voluntarily, but the subsequent series of events is almost entirely reflex action. In rapid succession food is placed in the mouth, thoroughly chewed and then placed on the tongue, ready to be swallowed. The tongue directs food through the upper throat, the pharynx rises, accepts the food and constricts to direct it to the sophagus where peristaltic action aided by gravity carries it to the stomach. Normal behavior in this process is that the respiratory functions are inhibited by reflex action; food is kept out of the nasal sinuses by elevation of the soft palate and out of the larynx by movement of the glottis and the epiglottis.

With swallowing dysfunction, the P/D patient can choke on food, liquids or saliva, especially if surprised by sudden noises or an unexpected touch. The possibility of inhaling food, drink or saliva is very much a fact of life for the Parkinsonian.

It is important that the caregiver and family members of a Parkinsonian know how to perform the Heimlich Maneuver to be used in the event of a choking episode. It is also highly recommended that family members be trained in CPR first aid for the safety of the family, including the Parkinsonian.

While there are a majority of Parkinsonians with excess saliva, there is a smaller group that has an opposing problem of having too little saliva. Too little saliva may be the result of mouth breathing, a side effect of medication.

Unlike excess saliva problems, a dry mouth usually can be relieved with chewing gum or sucking on a hard candy.

An excess of saliva can lead not only to choking but to drooling while awake or asleep. While awake it soon becomes a habit to keep a supply of handkerchiefs or tissues handy. While sleeping, you may want to spread a soft towel over your pillow and wear a sleep mask, as I do, to keep the eyes safe from nighttime irritation of saliva.

Teeth and Dental Care

The Parkinsonian is arriving at an age, usually, at which most of his contemporaries are having to devote more time, thought and money to the care and preservation of their teeth. However, the Parkinsonian is not subject to excessive dental problems.

Dental problems most commonly faced by the Parkinsonian are, in part, due to his P/D but they are also related to the aging process. One of the most troubling problems for the P/D patient is that he is doing less and less hard chewing, which eventually leads to gum disease and loose teeth. Add this problem to the loss or movement of teeth from causes other than P/D and you find the Parkinsonian developing a preference for soft foods, a slack jaw and a tendency to drool.

These problems are compounded by the patient's involuntary clenching of the muscles of the jaw, a circumstance which can occur while asleep, awake or engaged in some activity requiring intense concentration. Jaw clenching and teeth grinding (known technically as bruxism) are uncomfortable and destructive processes. Bruxism not only is deleterious to the teeth, it is a noisy and sometimes irritating sound which some spouses compare to raking one's fingernails across a blackboard.

This jaw clenching can have more than one unpleasant consequence. First, if it continues for an extended period it can result in tension-type headaches. Also, spasm-like jaw clenching while asleep can result in broken or chipped teeth.

Bruxism while asleep can, for the predominantly unilateral Parkinsonian, cause uneven wear and misalignment of teeth. If this clenching persists, whether awake or asleep, the patient should have his dentist provide him with a protective mouthpiece to be worn as needed to preserve and protect the teeth. These appliances are relatively inexpensive and can be worn during most activities, exercising included.

Blood Pressure

Most Parkinsonians find that if they have a problem with blood pressure it is with hypotension (low) rather than hypertension (high). There are many reasons why a patient with P/D may have blood pressure problems; not all of them are related to Parkinson's disease. The patient should not try to decide these things for himself but should confer with his physician and abide by his best judgment. However, the patient should be aware that some medicines prescribed for P/D can cause a substantial lowering of blood pressure.

For the Parkinsonian who finds that he has persistent or occasional low blood pressure, investigation may show that his hypotension may be drug related or due to other causes. Once the patient and his doctor decide the cause of the problem they can decide on a course of action.

Usually drug-related hypotension manifests itself with a lightheaded feeling on rising from bed or from a seated position. This lightheaded feeling may be the precursor of a faint, always a hazard for a person of mature years, especially when he has become more sedentary because of P/D. One thing that happens to the P/D patient after spending more time in bed or sitting is that blood pools in the legs. This is a result of varicosities in the veins of the lower extremities and a general loss of tone in the cardiovascular system.

Since the patient is already under instructions to exercise and be as active as his condition allows, the most frequent advice for the Parkinsonian is the use of elastic support hose. This can provide, for the Parkinsonian, a new lease on life judging from my own experience. These hose come in stockings and panty-hose styles and a variety of colors so that there should not be any reluctance by the patient to wear them should his doctor decide that they would be beneficial.

In my own case, I found that just about all of my exercise and mobility actions were easier and more positive and I felt safer on my feet when wearing the support hose. It is an effort to get them on and off, but that is a small price to pay for relief.

Cramps

Most Parkinsonians have had some experience with muscle cramps. These occur most frequently at night, and they most always affect the muscles of the leg, in the area of the gastrocnemius and the soleus muscles which comprise the major portion of the leg below and behind the knee. It has been my experience that cramps occur spontaneously, though I have triggered them by extending the foot beyond a comfortable limit while stretching. Almost all of my cramps affect the dominant, or preferred leg.

Once a cramp has been initiated, there is very little that can be done to relieve the condition. Vigorous massage is not recommended but firm pressure broadly applied may help alleviate the cramp. When able to move the affected part, it may be beneficial to move it through its complete range of motion several times and then apply heat in the form of a heating pad or a hot water bottle. Muscle soreness is almost always a post-cramping phenomenon best treated with more heat and light exercise.

If cramps are persistent or become a daily occurrence the Parkinsonian should consult with his physician to discuss the details of these cramping episodes and to determine whether any treatment is required.

Diet, Nutrition, Digestion and Elimination

In his search for a cure for his Parkinson's disease every Parkinsonian has, somewhere in his mind, the unvoiced idea that he might find a panacea which would not only arrest his disease but would reverse the symptoms as well. At present, it is a vain hope but one which almost everyone with whom I have talked admits having entertained at one time. First, it is exorbitant hopes for new medicines. Then, one turns to diet and, finally, to vitamins.

The vacuity of the simplistic approach to problem solution is demonstrated in a story

> *told about Thomas Edison, the great inventor and innovator. Though Edison was not trained or educated as a scientist or an engineer, his direct and often ingenuous approach to the practical solution of mechanical problems was widely admired and brought him great financial rewards. It seems, that in talking with a friend who happened to be a physician, Edison got interested in gout, its cause and cure. The story is not explicit as to whether Edison himself had gout, but given the period, his age, his affluence, and his work habits, he would have been a candidate. At any rate, he discovered from the doctor that gout was a collection of uric acid, usually in the first joint of the great toe, painful and disabling.*
>
> *"Ah ha" said Edison, the wizard of Menlo Park. "I have a laboratory with thousands of chemicals. We will take some samples of uric acid and apply various chemicals until we find one that will dissolve the uric acid and we have a cure. Simple." He tried but soon lost interest. Years later when Henry Ford moved the laboratory to Greenfield Village and Edison was an old man, there still was no cure for gout (Source uncertain).*

So much for simple solutions.

Food Cures

The Parkinsonian is hoping there is some way to help his disease through diet. He has done all that he and his doctor can do with medication. Why not try food?

He reads every book he can find on therapeutic diets and subscribes to health magazines. He learns how to lose weight with grapefruit, with gelatin desserts and with rice. But, he finds no way to lose Parkinson's disease. Just as there seems to be no great benefits to the Parkinsonian from dieting and vitamins there is no great harm in them either, unless grossly abused.

There have been a number of studies conducted concerning the supposition that a protein rich diet counteracted the beneficial effects of L-Dopa. Attempts to prove or disprove the theory have received more news coverage than they deserved. The results of the studies seem to confirm that any harm a high protein diet would cause would be minimal, so it is not a significant factor in present day treatment of Parkinson's disease.

There is some evidence that vitamin B6 which is included in many one-a-day vitamin supplements tends to counteract the beneficial effects of L-Dopa to some degree. It was a minor factor in earlier generations of L-Dopa but presently is not a matter of concern to the Parkinsonian. Here again, the patient's doctor is the best judge of that. Many physicians feel that vitamin supplements are not necessary but there are vitamin supplements available from which B6 has been eliminated.

The details of regulating protein intake, and the pro's and con's of vitamin supplements, and whether to take them, are beyond the scope of this book. There are excellent books on nutrition for further study if the patient or caregiver wants to pursue this fascinating subject further.

"The Complete Book of Nutrition," published by Dell and written by Cary and Steve Null, is a thorough no-nonsense guide which I have read with great interest. The Parkinsonian finds that, after a great deal of reading and study on the subject of his diet, he is at liberty to continue with any diet that suits his taste.

He should, however, take into consideration his own experience with side effects of medication in choosing the optimum time to take his medicine. In my own experience, I have found that, because of the relatively short "on" time of my medication, I do far better on four light meals a day instead of three heavier ones.

Alcohol Consumption and Smoking

This seems to be a good place to discuss P/D and the consumption of alcohol. Many physicians place such beverages off-limits for their P/D patients, not because they have been proven harmful but rather on the possibility that they might be harmful.

The case against alcohol, whether in the form of beer, wine or cocktails, is made on two bases. First, that the Parkinsonian should take nothing which might inhibit or detract from any of the medications being taken for his disease. Second, alcohol is a depressant and since depression is known to be a problem for Parkinsonians, alcohol should be avoided. These negative views of P/D and alcohol are not universally held and some physicians think that a modest amount of alcohol, one beer, one cocktail or a glass of wine is beneficial to the Parkinsonian, not a detriment. My own view on alcohol is to avoid it as a general rule but to allow an occasional festive drink.

Smoking is a habit that most people, whether Parkinsonian or not, wish they had never started. Though I have never smoked I am well aware of the hazards that smoking entails to Parkinsonians, as well as others. I also realize the physical and emotional needs smoking seems to satisfy for some individuals. If smoking is bad for the healthy individual, it can only be worse for the Parkinsonian. The loss of mobility, dexterity, flexibility and loss of lung capacity suffered by the P/D patient are burden enough without adding to the problem.

Advice: If you don't smoke now, don't start. If you smoke now, quit. And if you can't quit, at least cut down, and become familiar with tar and nicotine ratings and use the lowest you can tolerate.

Constipation

Another little understood effect of Parkinson's disease is in the peristalsis process in the alimentary canal. The peristalsis process is a wave-like motion of muscles in the intestinal walls which serves to move the contents of the duodenum through the small and large intestines. It is a reflex action normally, as is the action of the pyloric valve.

The P/D patient, as a result of diet, medication and deteriorating muscle control often finds himself with a problem of constipation.

Control of constipation in P/D is much the same as it is with average, healthy individuals over age 50. Bulk in the diet, sufficient liquid intake, giving up the notion that a daily bowel movement is the expected norm and a new determination that you are not going to let bowel habits rule your life should be sufficient. If constipation is persistent and does not respond to common sense habits and remedies, the next step is to consult with your doctor, taking care to determine that the physician is aware of the special needs and requirements of Parkinsonians.

Driving an Automobile

Driving an automobile safely is, at any age or any degree of disability, more a mental than a physical exercise. If the Parkinsonian was a good driver before the onset of the disease he will very likely continue to be a good driver. Conversely, if he was a marginal driver before, his illness may possibly rule him off the road far earlier than would be necessary for his physical short-comings alone.

One should remember that Parkinson's disease, while it causes tremor and disturbs motor functions, does not paralyze the patient. What is lost to P/D is facility of movement, not the ability to move.

The P/D patient usually finds that, in an emergency-type situation, he is capable of quick and positive movements. He also finds that he cannot sustain this emergency status for long periods of time. As to the tremor of P/D being a disabling factor, it should be remembered that the characteristic P/D tremor is present most often when the muscles are at rest. Muscle activity seems to mask the tremor so that the Parkinsonian is more comfortable doing something whether it be typing, wielding a paint brush, swinging a walking stick, or driving an automobile.

Driving is a Privilege

There is no way to establish how capable a driver has been, and presently is, other than through a subjective examination of the patient's driving record as compared with the ease and skill of his present performance. Giving up driving is such a traumatic point in one's life that few persons make the decision on their own, waiting instead to have the decision forced upon them by circumstances and the action of others.

It should be remembered that by the consent of the governed, the regulation of motor vehicle insurance, licensing and operation has been accepted as being for the good of the community. As such, one recognizes that driving is a privilege rather than a right.

There are many ways that a P/D patient can lose the privilege of being a licensed driver:

1) Voluntary surrender of license.
2) Revocation on failing state renewal examination.
3) Revocation by court for driving irresponsibly.
4) Revocation on recommendation of physician.
5) Refusal of license in new state of residence.

If the patient prepares himself mentally for a more deliberate driving pace and the additional care required in order to continue driving, he can extend his driving years considerably. Senior citizens groups in many cities offer a refresher driving course tailored for the older driver. Such a course can point out bad habits and driving problems which might otherwise have gone undetected.

Making Use of Special Parking Spaces

Many Parkinsonians shun the exercise of their right to use parking slots reserved for the disabled. Some drivers believe that the effort and expense of obtaining a distinctive license plate or decal is too much trouble. Others see it as an admission of their disability and shun the convenience as long as is possible.

It is an individual choice and should be left to the patient to decide. I feel that the distinctive license plate can serve as a safety device. The wheelchair symbol alerts other drivers that the P/D driver may take a little longer to maneuver.

In England, there used to be a requirement that novice drivers display on their automobiles a 10-inch square sign, with a white background and a large black, block letter "L" for learner. It served to alert the driving public to what might be a greater than normal road hazard. I think that our wheelchair symbol performs the same service.

Parkinsonians are urged to contact their state license authority for information about handicapped licensing.

Paraphernalia

As the patient's disease progresses and his symptoms worsen, the patient and the caregiver are constantly faced with coping difficulties in almost every facet of day-to-day living. Throughout this book I have mentioned several items which have helped me to cope or have alleviated the frustration that every Parkinsonian feels sooner or later. Here are some items I have found useful.

Carry with or keep handy:

A pill box with at least one day's medicine. I use one which resembles a fountain pen. It is metal and keeps medication handy and protected from light and moisture and is inconspicuous.

Visual aids, including spare glasses, lens cleaning tissues, a small magnifier and a lanyard to keep glasses handy when not in use, a small flashlight and nail clippers.

A ballpoint pen, a note pad, a small telephone amplifier and a spare hearing aid battery.

Getting in and out of clothes:

Hooks on a wall or door keep clothing and pajamas handy and visible.

A handy long-handled shoe horn, a back scratcher and a zipper puller, a convenient seat in the bathroom and a handy laundry hamper all serve to make life a little easier.

The use of velcro closures on shoes, outer wear and even sleep wear, are a great convenience, saving time and frustration.

The simple problem of snagging almost every garment I tried to put on with my watch, I solved by moving the watch to the opposite wrist. I have found that suspenders are more comfortable than a belt and I am more at ease since I began buying a larger size clothing, wearing everything a little looser. Mark Twain is reported to have said that old men have few comforts left besides comfortable shoes, loose clothing and a good cigar. I have no need for the cigar but I can endorse the rest of his list.

Morning Ablutions (or Whatever)

For the Parkinsonian there is always a great potential for inconvenience and frustration in the bathroom. One can't help remembering how swiftly one used to shave, shampoo and shower, and reflect on what a tedious chore those simple tasks have now become.

To relieve some of the tedium you need to do some planning and scheduling. Some of the tasks can be delayed until the medicine turns you "on". For the shower and bathtub, a seat in the tub can be reassuring and a hand-held shower can be safe and convenient. A sturdy towel rack can double as a handgrip for those unsteady moments as well as to keep towels at hand. A caddy to hold soap, shampoo and a long handled back scrubber can be useful in letting the Parkinsonian fend for himself much longer.

Other bathroom items of great convenience are: the elimination of childproof for medicine bottles; an electric toothbrush; an electric razor; a pressure-jet Water-Pik machine; pump-type toothpaste; soft packages for mouth wash; and mitt-type washcloths. Hair brushes and combs with large handles are available and are also a convenience.

As one grows older there never seems to be enough light in the bathroom, so I installed a new and brighter fixture. To further enhance the use of light, I installed on every available wall a number of 12" x 12" mirror tiles brightening the room considerably.

Exercises 14

There is an ongoing disagreement among those in the Parkinsonian community as to whether the stiff joints and weak muscles, which are symptoms of P/D, are a direct result of the disease or whether these symptoms are the result of disuse.

I choose to believe that these changes occur because of disuse and that the sooner one begins to exercise for flexibility, muscle strengthening and endurance, the better. I also believe that it is never too late to begin. Damage may have been done but reversal is possible though the benefits will never be 100 percent.

The thing that the Parkinsonian and the caregiver should keep in mind is that rehabilitation does not take place overnight. Increased flexibility, strength and endurance come slowly, but they do come if one is willing and diligent in their pursuit.

Logic tells us that flexibility comes before strength. Strength without flexibility creates a kind of paralysis of its own. So, a primary concern in an exercise program for a Parkinsonian should be to increase the range of motion of the joints before working on muscular strength.

The instituting of an exercise program for a Parkinsonian relies in great degree on the point at which the patient is starting. If he has been active in the past he may very well be able to start exercising at a higher intensity than the person who has been sedentary throughout his adult life. The judgment as to how strenuously a patient should exercise may need to be made by the physician or a physical therapist. However, the final arbiter of how much of what exercise is going to be the patient himself.

In the early stages of P/D, physical changes in the patient may not be obvious but the precursors are there. One sees the forward thrust of the head and neck, the rounded shoulders, an exaggeration of the curving of the spine, a forward tilt of the pelvis, bent knees, ankle and toe problems, as well as stiff shoulder joints, elbows and wrists, and unusual contortions of the hands and fingers. Though not as evident there is also a loss of flexibility of the ribcage.

An exercise program for Parkinsonians in the home (I am assuming that those in hospitals or other institutions will be attended by trained staff) does not require elaborate equipment. A clear space indoors, about 5' x 8' with a pad or a comforter, some light weights or substitute, a broomstick and a towel are all that are necessary to begin. Loose, comfortable clothing such as a warm-up or sweat suit makes exercise seem easier. Reasonably firm-soled shoes with sturdy uppers are preferable to exercising barefoot.

Before you begin exercising, a word of caution. There are countless numbers of exercise gurus extant today, each pushing his (or her) own version of the exercise game with video to match. Beware of the high-pressure sales pitch which promises too much too easily and at the other end of the spectrum, the masochist who says "make it hurt" or "no pain, no gain." Somewhere in the median there is a zone of sanity where the Parkinsonian can find flexibility and strength without doing irreparable harm to his body and spirit.

Flexibility Exercises

1. Stretch out full length on your mat, supine (on your back), and try to stretch your body to full reach. Keep your elbows straight, arms close to your sides. The top of your head should reach for one wall and the tips of your toes should reach for the other. Try to touch the back of your knees, the small of your back and the nape of your neck to the mat. Stretch 15 seconds, relax 30 seconds, repeat 5 cycles to start.

2. Turn over and stretch out prone (on your stomach). Repeat the above exercise with 5 each stretch and relaxation cycles. Keep arms at sides and turn head to left or right, whichever is most comfortable.

3. Stand and face the wall, the tips of your toes about 1 foot from the wall. With palms about shoulder height and touching the wall, lean forward until your forehead touches the wall. Support yourself by pushing against the wall while rising on tiptoe, then walk or slide your palms up the wall as far as you can reach. Keep the legs and spine as erect as possible. Walk palms down to shoulder height, relax 30 seconds and repeat 5 cycles. Increase repetitions as you grow stronger and more flexible.

4. Seated or standing, drape a towel around your neck. Grasp the towel with both hands, keeping them as close together as is comfortable. Holding the spine as erect as is possible, raise the arms as high above the head as far as is possible. Begin with 5 repetitions; increase as you feel stronger.

5. While standing or sitting, fold arms with hands to elbow, upper arms held parallel to the floor. Holding this position, twist the upper torso as far left as is comfortable. Hold this position for two beats. Return to center position. Repeat by going to the right. Return to center. Repeat 5 cycles and increase as you grow stronger.

As a supplement or as an alternate to the previous exercise, assume the same arm position and, while seated, try to touch the elbow to the opposite knee. Right elbow to left knee, left elbow to right knee. Repeat for 5 cycles, increasing as you feel stronger.

6. Seated on the floor, keep the spine as straight as possible. Hold one leg with knee comfortably bent; the other leg extended to the front resting on a large book, pillow or block, enough to riase the heels 3" to 4" off the floor. Lean forward until you feel discomfort. Try to touch the right toe with the left hand, the left toe with the right hand. Do 5 repetitions to start, adding repetitions as you grow stronger.

7. Lie on your back on the floor, holding arms out straight and clear of the mat. Stretching arms to full length, move hands in circles about 6 inches in diameter. Do 5 circles clockwise, then 5 circles counterclockwise. Repeat for 5 repetitions. Perform the same cycles with each leg separately, knee straight and toes extended with the leg lifted clear of the mat. Repeat with other leg, making 5 cycles for each.

8. Stand with feet shoulder width apart, spine as straight as possible, head stretched toward the ceiling. Raise both arms to the side to shoulder height with elbows as straight as possible, fingertips extended. Raise arms above the head, touch fingertips together if possible. Return to previous position. Swing arms from side to front at shoulder height, touch palms if possible. Return extended arms to side. Touch shoulders with finger-tips. Keeping elbows at shoulder height, attempt to touch elbows together behind your back. Drop arms to sides, shake to relax. Repeat each exercise 5 repetitions. Increase as you grow stronger.

9. Most Parkinsonians have a "head-set" problem which results from involuntary constrictions of the muscles which regulate and control the positioning of the head. The result is that the Parkinsonian often has posture headaches and has the feeling that the vertebrae in his neck are "grinding" together. Exercises of the head and neck should begin with range of movement.

Without force, tilt head forward chin on chest 5 times. Then tilt head back, chin up 5 times. Next, tilt head left, ear on shoulder, head right, ear on shoulder. Do each exercise 5 times.

Then, rotate head in a circle 5 revolutions clockwise and 5 counterclockwise. Next, ring an imaginary doorbell with your chin thrusting forward as far as possible 10 times, tucking chin to chest after each thrust.

10. Exercises of the forearm, wrist and hand can take many forms but nothing exotic is called for in the case of the Parkinsonian. Raise arms to shoulder height and to the side, hands open and palms down. Rotate wrists to turn palms up, then back to palms down. Repeat 10 times. This movement is called pronation and is a movement many Parkinsonians do not realize they are losing. Repeat pronation 10 times with arms held forward at shoulder height. Drop arms and shake out then resume previous posture. Repeat side and front pronation exercises while aggressively making and releasing a fist with both hands, 10 each, side and front.

11. Exercises for the fingers can usually be the patient's choice because the variety of dexterity exercises is as endless as the variety of symptoms displayed by Parkinsonians. Using a typewriter or playing the piano, or a simulation of such exercises, can provide the variety of experience and the repetitive actions necessary for keeping the hands supple and fit. Model building or calligraphy, painting or sketching, needlepoint, and puppetry are only a few of the ways Parkinsonians cajole their errant fingers into doing their duty. A good thing to remember is that most of Parkinsonian tremor is "resting tremor". Hands that are always occupied have far less tremor, as a rule.

After a reasonably good degree of flexibility has been reached (one to two weeks) the Parkinsonian can begin cautiously adding strength exercises to his program, assuming the patient feels comfortable wit his progress in the flexibility phase.

Strength Exercises

The first thing to remember in beginning strength exercises is that the flexibility exercises, at a high number of repetitions, should be continued. Strength, while important, should always be secondary.

Exercising successfully for strength can be more precise and effective if one takes the time to learn the proper terminology for the muscles you are exercising: the deltoids, biceps and triceps in the arms; the pectorals, latissimus and gluteus of the trunk; and the biceps, quadriceps and gastrocnemius in the leg to name a few. It also requires a small amount of equipment to achieve best results. A padded pressing bench with a leg exercise arm at one end and a tilt section and a bar-bell rack is the most useful tool, next to weights. A beginner's set of weights with a total weight of 80 to 120 pounds is usually sufficient. A set with one long bar with collars and two short bars with collars (barbell and dumbbell respectively) plus an assortment of weights is all that is needed.

Before beginning to train with weights take a few minutes to go through some flexibility exercises of your choosing. Five to 10 minutes is sufficient. Then, get on the bench and begin.

1. Start on the bench in the prone position, working on the legs with minimum weight, lifting from the heel. This strengthens the biceps muscles in the back of the thigh. Do 5 repetitions, rest, do 5 more, rest, and do 5 more. Turn to a supine position (on your back) and lift straight leg with minimum weight. This strengthens the quadriceps in the front of the thigh. Do the same repetitions and pattern as in the prone position.

2. In the supine position, do alternate leg lifts bending the knee slightly if the pull on abdominals is too great. Do three sets of 5 with each leg. Repeat in the prone position, lifting straight leg. Bend the knee if the gluteal muscles of the posterior and the latissimus muscles of the lower back feel strained. Do three sets of 5 in the same pattern.

3. Weight training for the torso and arms may be while standing or may be done in a sitting position, using a low backless stool or bench. For the Parkinsonian, the aim is not to become a body builder or muscle man. The routines used should be discussed with the physician and an experienced physical therapist.

A word of caution: While the Parkinsonian is advised to consult with his physician before beginning any exercise program, it is even more important that strength exercises be done with the knowledge and advice of a medical professional. Otherwise, the patient may exceed limits placed on him by the advance of P/D. If at all possible, any exercise-for-strength program should be reviewed by the patient's physician or a physical therapist prior to its initiation.

Where To Get Help 15

The patient, the caregiver, family and concerned friends always have unanswered questions relating to Parkinson's disease, questions in more detail than the physician can anticipate or has time to answer. Where to turn for answers then?

First, to the national organizations who deal with P/D specifically. These groups have information available in newsletters and pamphlets concerning the latest developments in research projects, new treatment and medication, reports from and schedules for the many symposia being held related to Parkinson's disease, and providing hints on living with P/D.

A cautionary word about national organizations for P/D. There is not just one organization, but several. In my opinion this is unfortunate because it splinters the support for research on the disease. I am not going to say that there is antagonism among these organizations but the reader should not be surprised if there is a hint of acrimony displayed in this area. For example, I was interrupted during a television interview by a representative of one group when I cited estimates of the number of Parkinsonians from other groups.

Getting Help Locally

Though it is good to make use of the resources of national groups, in my opinion a more direct and personal source for information and support for the Parkinsonian is the local Parkinson's disease support group. The help received is personal and to the point because it is given by persons who are living with P/D and who have already fought many of the battles a recently diagnosed patient is just beginning to face. Almost every metropolitan area has a support group and inquiries are always welcome.

Whether you are a patient just beginning to face the problems of living with P/D, one who has been isolated and believes that he alone is struggling with the disease, or just have unanswered questions about life with P/D, you are urged to contact your local support group. The patient, and caregiver, will be advised about mailing lists, counseling arrangements, invited to attend meetings and asked to participate in other activities.

The Lone Parkinsonian

The Parkinson's disease patient who lives alone is in particular need of the companionship, support and guidance found in these groups. The lone Parkinsonian has ample time to feel solitary and alone. The mere knowledge that the support group exists is comforting.

Most support groups have some sort of networking arrangement, formal or informal, by means of which lone and isolated patients are kept in the mainstream with visits, telephone calls and expressions of genuine concern.

I have been referring to the P/D patient who is physically alone, without a spouse, relative or caregiver living in the same household. This is a difficult situation and requires all the ingenuity one can muster to cope with the symptoms and the uncertainties of the disease without reinforcement and support.

There is, however, another lone P/D patient one encounters all too often. This is the Parkinsonian who has a spouse or live-in relative who is physically or emotionally incapable of acting as a caregiver, who refuses for whatever reason, to involve himself with helping the Parkinsonian cope with his disease.

There are many persons of this description who refuse to accept the reality of the Parkinsonian's medical problems. The fact is, there are some apparently healthy adults who cannot handle illness and stress. For that reason, we can only feel sympathy for them. This, however, does not change our primary concern for the P/D patient who is in need of help just as surely as though he lived alone.

For these patients, then, their only recourse in the absence of a caregiver is to go it alone, establishing their own network of support, attending and participating in support group activities and making use of the experience of others with the same problems or with an understanding of these problems. This is not to say that the lone Parkinsonian is going to have it easy. Far from it. It is very hard to cope alone, but it can, and is, being done.

The Patient and Caregiver as a Team

Many support groups for other diseases discourage the patient from attending their meetings, tailoring programs toward the spouse or caregiver. This is not done in the

Parkinson's disease support groups. With P/D, the patient and spouse are considered a team. They are encouraged to attend and to participate as partners.

Parkinson's disease support group meetings can be a real challenge at times with many patients attending who have communication difficulties yet have something important to say. Often, when handed a microphone, they will find the words, the breath and the clarity of diction necessary to get the message across. In other cases, when it is obvious that the message is not getting through, the caregiver or spouse will diplomatically step in to translate.

There are a great number of support groups for Parkinson's disease, mostly centered in metropolitan population hubs. Even though it is necessary for some Parkinsonians to travel some distance they find that it is worth the drive. The amount of organization and bureaucracy in support groups varies widely as does the type and the quality of their programs. What needs to be kept in mind is that these groups are made up of volunteers, many of whom are P/D patients themselves. As such, they should be given a wide latitude in attendance, abilities and attitude.

Organizing and Sustaining a Support Group

The chief problem in organizing and sustaining a support group is getting people involved and making a contribution by working for the good health of the organization. The many tasks involved with making a group run smoothly all too often falls to the same overworked volunteers who arrange for meeting space, PA system, name tags, notices of meetings in the media, newsletters, publicity, programs and speakers, refreshments and cleanup after meetings.

Far too many patients and family members expect to come to the meetings, be enlightened and informed and go home, giving no thought or help toward making the wheels go around. Support groups need active and supportive members.

One group has a motto, "Do something! Either lead, follow or get out of the way!" That says it.

Addresses for National Groups

Here are the addresses of some of the national organizations which can be of help to the patient and the Parkinsonian family:

The American Parkinson Disease Association
116 John Street
New York, NY 10038

United Parkinson Foundation
360 West Superior Street
Chicago, IL 60610

PEP.USA
Parkinson's Educational Program
1800 Park Newport #302
Newport Beach, CA 92660

Parkinson's Disease Foundation
William Black Medical Research Building
Columbia Presbyterian Medical Center
650 West 168th Street
New York, NY 10032

Parkinson's Support Groups of America
1707 Old Stage Road
Alexandria, VA 22308

Convenience products and accessories for the P/D patient can be bought at many local medical supply outlets. Sears has a Hospital/Sickroom catalog which is available on request. A mail-order supplier I have ordered from is Dr. Leonard's Health Care Products, 74-20th Street, Brooklyn, NY 11232.

The U.S. Consumer Information Center of the General Services Administration, Box 100, Peublo, CO 81002 has a number of health-related publications available at reasonable costs. Many are free.

For travelers, the Airport Operators Council International, 1700 K Street N.W., Washington, DC 20006 has a publication showing airport access provisions for the handicapped in some detail worldwide. The Itinerary Magazine is devoted to travelers with handicaps. It publishes six times a year from P.O. Box 1084, Bayonne, NJ 07002.

Do's And Don'ts 16

As with most problems one has to face as an adult, one soon develops a list of things he wishes others would or, as is the more frequent case, wouldn't do! This is no less true with Parkinson's disease regardless of whether one is the patient or the caregiver. I have compiled a list of pet peeves and irritants of typical couples who have lived with the realities of Parkinson's disease for a number of years.

These comments are directed to: (1) the patient and caregiver; (2) the patient; and, (3) the caregiver. Some may seem too trivial to mention but, remember, one man's trivia is another man's philosophy. Other comments may seem too harsh. The thought here is that we are adults dealing with adult problems and we waste valuable time and energy when we refuse to face reality.

FOR THE PATIENT AND THE CAREGIVER

Don't isolate yourselves. Both parties will profit by continuing a near-normal social life.

Don't be a bore. The world does not revolve around your disease. After the initial announcement, comment to others sparingly. Go into detail only if asked and stop when they begin to fidget.

Keep your preoccupation within reason. Do not assume that others and their families always enjoy good health. One's P/D may seem trivial to a person with terminal cancer or to someone with a spouse far along with Alzheimer's disease.

Don't expect too much from family and friends. The way to have a friend is to continue with the give-and-take of friendship. To have a friend, be a friend.

Give each other some time and space to be alone. Too much togetherness is as bad as too little. This right to be alone should apply to interrogation as well. If a person has been out, don't demand, "Where have you been?" Let the individual feel that he is free to explain or not.

Household chores and activities should be shared after an adult discussion of work sharing. Don't assume that the spouse automatically knows what needs to be done or knows how to do an unfamiliar task.

Don't disagree at length in the company of others. If one spouse is telling a story don't interject. Allow for variations in details of a story.

Be civil to each other. It is important at any time but much more so with an illness.

Be honest with each other. Life is too short to have to constantly be asking oneself, "I wonder what she meant by that?"

FOR THE CAREGIVER

Don't coddle the patient; don't hover.

Don't finish a sentence for the patient.

Don't answer a question obviously intended for the patient.

Don't talk to others about the patient as though he was not present.

Don't make an invalid of the patient by becoming a "gopher". Let the patient get up and get his snack even if you can do it faster and better.

Don't be oversolicitous.

Don't discourage the patient when he proposes a new project or activity, better to try and fail than to refuse to take a chance.

Do be on the alert for hazards to the patient in his home environment. An inconveniently placed chair or table or a throw rug which bunches up is all it takes to turn a functioning Parkinsonian into an invalid.

Be flexible. There is no law that says that bedtime is 11:00 p.m. or that lunch is at noon.

Do insist that you have time of your own to do nothing or to do your own thing.

Do not lose your own identity by becoming an adjunct or an extension of the patient. Take time to be yourself.

Do help with a coat sleeve or a door if it can be done in an unobtrusive way.

Do encourage the patient to try new hobbies, pursue new ideas and health initiatives, and do remember to do the same thing for yourself.

FOR THE PATIENT

Don't be a complainer. Try to keep a positive attitude.

Don't assume that a casual conversation calls for a complete recital of your medical condition, your medication and dosages.

Don't assume that the stranger on the street or the highway will make an allowance for your disability. He may think that you are deliberately trying to inconvenience him. Don't be stubborn about right-of-way and such civilities. Give way and appear magnanimous.

Do try to stay active, mentally and physically.

Do work on your diction and speaking volume.

Don't rely on your spouse to be both ears and a mouthpiece for you when it is only a convenience and not a necessity.

Parkinson's Disease: One Man's Chronology 17

The following chronology is a personal one and as such should not be considered typical or atypical. It is merely representative of the progressive nature of the disease as it has affected me.

Year 1, 1971:

I had the first sign of symptoms. I began to switch my keys to my right pocket from my left (I am left-handed) as it became easier to unlock the car with my right hand. My watch on my right wrist began to get in my way so I moved it to my left wrist. In closing a field office I noticed, in lifting storage files, that my left arm, especially the elbow, felt weak. I began having some trouble with writing. The size of the script got smaller and it was tiring to write for any length of time. I did not consult a doctor about the problems which I felt were related to traumatic arthritis from a broken elbow suffered in the Army in 1943.

Year 2, 1972:

I changed jobs, leaving an employer of 17 years, a traumatic experience at age 49. I began to have "tennis elbow" pains in my left elbow. My handwriting continued to be more difficult, smaller and less intelligible. I noticed that my left arm and hand shivered uncontrollable in cold weather.

My left leg seemed to be puffy and heavy, and it dragged a little -- especially when I was tired. That was not new. For I had experienced problems with that leg after having phlebitis following a long illness with pleurisy when I was in my early 20s. I still did not consult a doctor about my problems.

Year 3, 1973:

It continued to become more difficult to use the left arm and hand. Strength and dexterity continued to decrease, writing grew more difficult to initiate and to continue for any length of time. The left leg continued to feel heavy and draggy; the left foot seemed prone to drop, causing a tripping hazard. An EKG during a routine physical gave unusual traces for the left extremities. Discussion with my family doctor agreed with my arthritis/phlebitis scenario.

Year 4, 1974:

Back to the family doctor, same problem. He sent me for an X-ray of the painful elbow. The observant radiologist urged me to have my doctor send me to a neurologist. My family doctor set it up. The neurologist took 20 minutes to make the diagnosis. He had me walk, turn, stand on one foot, touch my nose, button my shirt, smile, grimace and bring samples of earlier handwriting. He was not forthcoming about prognosis or treatment.

He sent me to several diagnostic centers, confirming his diagnosis and screening for the elimination of other diseases, epilepsy, brain tumor or anything else which might be masquerading as P/D. This required several visits over a week or more.

He began my medication with 2 mg of Artane three times a day. That was later increased to 5 mg and then stopped when I became nauseated after every dose. He switched me to Sinemet 10/100 three per day plus one Symmetrel 100 mg, later going to four Sinemet 10/100 per day. I continued on this dosage for the rest of the year doing very well, with my symptoms relieved almost entirely. I was successful in a dispute with FAA to keep my pilot's license and I continued to fly.

Year 5, 1975:

Medication continued to be quite effective and my condition did not change appreciably, no tremor or dyskinesia. My major complaint was that I tired easily and more frequently.

My problem was compounded by the heavy travel and long hours my work entailed.

Year 6, 1976:

A busy year with business travel very heavy. Slow movements and fatigue were my main problems. Sinemet dosage increased to 25/250, 3 per day; Symmetrel 100 mg, 2 per day. I stayed fit with vigorous walking, using a cane or staff to swing for help in establishing rhythm. Still played tennis but poorly.

Year 7, 1977:

I had a bad year. Work was more demanding with heavy travel in a firm grown more youth oriented. Adding to the strain was the illness and death of my mother-in-law and a long bout with a recurrent eye disease (not related to P/D). Additionally, my wife had spinal surgery. Medication was increased to 4 Sinemet 25/250 and 2 Symmetrel 100 mg. I experienced fatigue, a low tolerance to cold, a loss of dexterity, dragging my left foot when tired, and a loss of volume and clarity in speaking became more noticeable. I still looked and acted quite normal, and I had a difficult time convincing my company management that I needed to slow my pace of work. At last, I took the initiative and asked for a six-month leave of absence. This time off gave me an opportunity to work on physical fitness and to re-establish my emotional health.

Year 8, 1978:

I went back to work with the understanding that I would limit my travel and do only one project at a time with an opportunity to take time off between projects. Parkinson's disease symptoms stayed relatively level and dosages of medications remained stable throughout the year. I continued my exercise program, walking and jogging, and some swimming. My fatigue and tripping hazard of dragging my left foot stayed about the same.

Year 9, 1979:

P/D symptoms remained stable with no changes in medication or in dosages. I spent three months in the New York office and worked long hours with an understanding client. I made trips to the Soviet Union and the Kentucky Derby. Lack of stamina was my major complaint.

Year 10, 1980:

I did three short projects and still had three months off. My condition was stable, with no change in symptoms, medication or dosages.

Year 11, 1981:

I continued working at a reduced pace, and gave up driving a stickshift car for an automatic. I bought a canoe and a home computer for physical and mental exercise and recreation. My symptoms were stable and medication unchanged but I did notice more abrupt "on-off" phenomena which made me more conscious of the disease.

Year 12, 1982:

I bought a retirement home and began to make detailed plans for retirement. I worked all year at relatively low tempo. No great change occurred in type or severity of symptoms or medication. I continued physical and mental exercises.

Year 13, 1983:

I continued working at slowed pace, but made firm plans to retire on my 61st birthday, February 11, 1984. I became associated with Parkinson's disease research program of Cole Neuroscience Foundation and my present neurologist at University of Tennessee Medical Center in Knoxville.

I had to undergo a six-week duration, partial drug holiday. I was unable to work during this time but it was not necessary to be hospitalized. I began a new regimen of medication: Sinemet 25/250, 3 per day; Symmetrel 100 mg, 2 per day; and Parlodel 2.5 mg, 3 per day. Later in the year, the Parlodel was increased to 5 mg, 3 per day, with good results.

Year 14, 1984:

I had my first pronounced decremental decrease in capabilities due to death of my mother and changes related to retirement. Nightmares and anxiety dreams increased in frequency and severity. I was given Sinequan 10 mg to aid with sleep problems. Walking increased in difficulty. I maintained three-mile distance but due to shorter pace and fatigue the distance formerly covered in 45 minutes now took an hour. Bicycling continued with 10 miles or more on straight and level roads, continued to do five miles in my kayak without difficulty.

Year 15, 1985:

My adjustment to retirement was surprisingly free of problems. Physical conditioning continued well with little noticeable decrement in any area of activity. I had a slight problem with impotence but worked it out satisfactorily with spouse and advice from my physician.

Year 16, 1986:

I continued on the same medicine and with the same exercise program. I lost some ground during the year due to concern over the breakup of the marriage of my oldest child. I gradually worked out of my depression over family problems.

Year 17, 1987:

No changes occurred in routine or medication. It was increasingly more difficult to get sufficient exercise, especially in cold weather. I continued to write, trying to do 1,000 words per day, two hours at the typewriter. My proficiency with the kayak, bicycle and driving a car were still virtually undiminished though requiring more care.

Year 18, 1988:

Fatigue, stiffness and increasing full-body tremor present a problem for physical conditioning but I continued trying. Physical losses were compensated for by a continued highly satisfactory state of mental health and attitude. I passed my 65th birthday milestone without any emotional upset.

Year 19, 1989:

I continue to be intellectually active, but I have lost some ground physically. My "off" periods are more severe. I am using a cane more often; festination is an almost constant problem and I have begun using a walker in "off" periods. An attempt to modify and improve medication mix, dosage and intervals was not successful and my doctor returned me to the medication routine which has been in effect for the last five years. I am more restless during sleep. I still mow the grass and walk, but fatigue is more noticeable. I am better able to concentrate and perform more demanding activities in the morning hours. My spirits are still good. I am looking forward to every new day and to many happy and useful years ahead.

POSTSCRIPT

It is my intention to revise and reissue this book as time passes and my Parkinson's disease symptoms worsen. I hope, at the same time, to be able to report new and exciting developments in Parkinson's disease research.

In order to make a new edition as interesting and as factual as possible I welcome letters from Parkinsonians and caregivers. Write me and relate any antedotes or helpful hints you think would be of interest to others and which you are willing to share.

Address correspondence to:

Jon Robert Pierce
Parkinsonian
P.O. Box 3204
Oak Ridge, TN 37832

Late Breaking News

As we go to press, the search goes on to find better medications for P/D and to eventually find means to arrest, prevent and cure the disease. The recent approval by the United States Food and Drug Administration for the use of

Deprenyl in the treatment of Parkinson's disease was welcome news for members of the Parkinsonian community.

Deprenyl has been in use in Europe for an adjunct to Sinemet therapy for about 10 years. It has been used primarily to smooth out the "off-on" stages which become more troublesome as Sinemet loses some of its efficacy after protracted use. Deprenyl is not expected to be useful for all Parkinsonians but the possibility should be discussed with the patient's physician.

Deprenyl will be marketed under the name of Elderpryl and others as licensees for the Hungarian originators.

Appendix

Parkinson's Incapacity Evaluation

It's Easy As Pie!

How it works:

> *Think of yourself when you were at your best. Call that 100. Do this for all three categories: mobility, communication and cognition. The average of these (A + B + C/3) is your base, which is 100. Being honest with yourself, judge your disability in each category. "A" is how well you get around; "B" is how well you understand and how well you are understood on the telephone, or in conversation. "C" is how well you think, remember, and/or handle abstract thought.*

A -- Mobility Factor:

Use of cane = 90; festination = 75; use of walker = 60; use of wheelchair = 40; bedridden = 20; bedridden, moving with assistance = 20.

B -- Communication Factor:

Loss of volume = 90; loss of intellegibility = 70; unable to use telephone = 50; incomprehensible to strangers = 40; incomprehensible to spouse = 20; unable to communicate in any fashion = 10.

C -- Cognition Factor:

Forgets to take medicine = 90; stops intellectual pursuits, reading = 75; loss of train of thought, interest in community = 50; neglects personal health, hygiene = 30; apathy and lack of interest in self and family, complete detachment = 10.

Calculations:

Enter your present Mobility number (0 to 100) in "A"
Enter your present Communication number (0 to 100) in "B"
Enter your present Cognition number (0 to 100) in "C"

A -- Mobility: _____
B -- Communication: _____
C -- Cognition: _____

Add A,B and C. Then, divide the results by 3. This is your PIE Factor.

Current PIE Factor:____
Date Calculated: ____

(Save for future reference. Extra PIE calculation forms are at the end of this chapter. Copy these and use to track the progression of your disease.)

Some of the Symptoms

(No one patient is likely to have all of these symptoms and no one symptom is an indication or confirmation of P/D.)

Symptoms and Manifestations

Balance: Falling, awkward movements, vertigo
Cramps: Of the arms, legs and/or entire body
Dexterity: Handwriting loss, clumsiness
Elimination: Incontinence, constipation
Eyes: Slow blink rate, poor visual field
Facial changes: Expressionless, mask-like, little smile
Faintness: When rising from the bed or a chair
Freezing: Unable to initiate movements
Jaws: Clinching, grinding of teeth
Mental: Depression, personality changes
Posture: Rounded shoulders, head thrust forward
Sleep: Disturbed, nightmares, anxiety
Slow movement: May/may not involve whole body
Speech: Low, monotone, unintelligible
Stiff joints: Flexibility, movement range loss
Throat: Trouble swallowing, choking, drooling
Tremor: Resting tremor or palsy of hand(s)

Useful Medications

Following is a partial list of medications used to treat P/D. Some of these drugs are useful in treatment of other ailments, as well.

Classification/ Trade Name	Generic Name	Form and Dosage
Antihistamines		
Benadryl	Diphenhydramine	Tablets 25,25 mg Capsule 25,50 mg Liquid 12.5 mg/5 ml
Anticholinergics		
Cogentin	Benztropine	Tablets 0.5,1,2 mg
Akineton	Biperiden	Tablets 2 mg
Parsidol	Ethopropazine	Tablets 10,50 mg
Disipal	Orphenadrine	Tablets 50 mg
Norflex	Orphenadrine	Tablets 100 mg E/R
Norgesic*		
Kemadrin	Procyclidine	Tablets 5 mg
Artane	Trihexyphenidyl	Tablets 2,5 mg
Tremin		
Dopamine Agonist		
Parlodel	Bromocriptine	Tablets 2.5 mg Capsule 5 mg
Dopamine Precursors		
Dopar	Levodopa	Capsule 100,250,500 mg
Larodopa	Levodopa	Capsule 100,250,500 mg
Modopar**	Benserazide Levodopa	Not available in U.S.
Sinemet**	Carbidopa Levodopa	Tablets 10/100 mg Tablets 25/100 mg Tablets 25/250 mg
Lodosyn**	Carbidopa	Tablets 25 mg
Miscellaneous		
Symmetrel	Amantadine	Tablets 100 mg Capsule 100 mg Liquid 50 mg/5 ml
Deprenyl***	Jumex Eldepryl	No information

*Combined with Aspirin and Caffeine

**These are Peripheral Decarboxylase Inhibitors. They may decrease side effects of Levodopa.

***This drug has been experimental, but was approved for use by patients whose doctors recommend it as of July 1989.

Cost of Medication and Treatment

Note: It is rare to find two Parkinsonians who have the same story to tell, who followed the same path to diagnosis and treatment or who are taking identical medication in identical amounts. However, the recently diagnosed Parkinsonian needs an idea of the costs which apply to treatment of his disease.

Maintenance care by the physician on a continuing basis will apply after diagnosis and stabilization, and usually will involve two to four office visits a year. The cost of each visit is $30 to $70, for an annual cost of $80 to $250. Initial costs of diagnosis and confirmation of diagnosis are approximately $100 and $400, respectively.

Medication costs vary widely. First, the P/D patient should not expect to find generic equivalents for his medication. For the most part, they don't exist. Markups for the same medicine will vary from one pharmacy to the next and shopping around may yield considerable savings.

In my own medication routine I take three drugs:

Sinimet: 25/250 mg at $0.53 each, 3-1/3 per day =	$1.87
Parlodel: 5 mg at $1.58 each, 3 per day =	4.74
Symmetrel: 100 mg at $0.60 each, 2 per day =	1.20
Cost per day (as of December 31, 1988):	$6.81
Cost per annum (as of December 31, 1988):	$2,485.65

Parkinson's Incapacity Evaluation

(A) Mobility Factor: Use of cane = 90; festination = 75; use of walker = 60; use of wheelchair = 40; bedridden = 20; bedridden, moving with assistance = 20.

(B) Communication Factor: Loss of volume = 90; loss of intellegibility = 70; unable to use telephone = 50; incomprehensible to strangers = 40; incomprehensible to spouse = 20; unable to communicate in any fashion = 10.

(C) Cognition Factor: Forgets to take medicine = 90; stops intellectual pursuits, reading = 75; loss of train of thought, interest in community = 50; neglects personal health, hygiene = 30; apathy and lack of interest in self and family, complete detachment = 10.

To calculate, enter your present mobility score in A. Enter your present communication score in B, and your present cognition score in C. Add and divide by 3. This is your PIE Factor.

A:Mobility = _____
B:Communication = _____
C:Cognition = _____

Date Calculated:__________
PIE Factor:__________

Previous Date Calculated:__________
Previous PIE Factor:__________
Change in PIE Factor: (Previous-Current):__________

Parkinson's Incapacity Evaluation

(A) Mobility Factor: Use of cane = 90; festination = 75; use of walker = 60; use of wheelchair = 40; bedridden = 20; bedridden, moving with assistance = 20.

(B) Communication Factor: Loss of volume = 90; loss of intellegibility = 70; unable to use telephone = 50; incomprehensible to strangers = 40; incomprehensible to spouse = 20; unable to communicate in any fashion = 10.

(C) Cognition Factor: Forgets to take medicine = 90; stops intellectual pursuits, reading = 75; loss of train of thought, interest in community = 50; neglects personal health, hygiene = 30; apathy and lack of interest in self and family, complete detachment = 10.

To calculate, enter your present mobility score in A. Enter your present communication score in B, and your present cognition score in C. Add and divide by 3. This is your PIE Factor.

A:Mobility = _____
B:Communication = _____
C:Cognition = _____

Date Calculated:__________
PIE Factor:__________

Previous Date Calculated:__________
Previous PIE Factor:__________
Change in PIE Factor: (Previous-Current):__________

Parkinson's Incapacity Evaluation

(A) Mobility Factor: Use of cane = 90; festination = 75; use of walker = 60; use of wheelchair = 40; bedridden = 20; bedridden, moving with assistance = 20.

(B) Communication Factor: Loss of volume = 90; loss of intellegibility = 70; unable to use telephone = 50; incomprehensible to strangers = 40; incomprehensible to spouse = 20; unable to communicate in any fashion = 10.

(C) Cognition Factor: Forgets to take medicine = 90; stops intellectual pursuits, reading = 75; loss of train of thought, interest in community = 50; neglects personal health, hygiene = 30; apathy and lack of interest in self and family, complete detachment = 10.

To calculate, enter your present mobility score in A. Enter your present communication score in B, and your present cognition score in C. Add and divide by 3. This is your PIE Factor.

A:Mobility = _____
B:Communication = _____
C:Cognition = _____

Date Calculated:__________
PIE Factor:__________

Previous Date Calculated:__________
Previous PIE Factor:__________
Change in PIE Factor: (Previous-Current):__________

Parkinson's Incapacity Evaluation

(A) Mobility Factor: Use of cane = 90; festination = 75; use of walker = 60; use of wheelchair = 40; bedridden = 20; bedridden, moving with assistance = 20.

(B) Communication Factor: Loss of volume = 90; loss of intellegibility = 70; unable to use telephone = 50; incomprehensible to strangers = 40; incomprehensible to spouse = 20; unable to communicate in any fashion = 10.

(C) Cognition Factor: Forgets to take medicine = 90; stops intellectual pursuits, reading = 75; loss of train of thought, interest in community = 50; neglects personal health, hygiene = 30; apathy and lack of interest in self and family, complete detachment = 10.

To calculate, enter your present mobility score in A. Enter your present communication score in B, and your present cognition score in C. Add and divide by 3. This is your PIE Factor.

A:Mobility = _____
B:Communication = _____
C:Cognition = _____

Date Calculated:__________
PIE Factor:__________

Previous Date Calculated:__________
Previous PIE Factor:__________
Change in PIE Factor: (Previous-Current):__________

Parkinson's Incapacity Evaluation

(A) Mobility Factor: Use of cane = 90; festination = 75; use of walker = 60; use of wheelchair = 40; bedridden = 20; bedridden, moving with assistance = 20.

(B) Communication Factor: Loss of volume = 90; loss of intellegibility = 70; unable to use telephone = 50; incomprehensible to strangers = 40; incomprehensible to spouse = 20; unable to communicate in any fashion = 10.

(C) Cognition Factor: Forgets to take medicine = 90; stops intellectual pursuits, reading = 75; loss of train of thought, interest in community = 50; neglects personal health, hygiene = 30; apathy and lack of interest in self and family, complete detachment = 10.

To calculate, enter your present mobility score in A. Enter your present communication score in B, and your present cognition score in C. Add and divide by 3. This is your PIE Factor.

A:Mobility = _____
B:Communication = _____
C:Cognition = _____

Date Calculated:__________
PIE Factor:__________

Previous Date Calculated:__________
Previous PIE Factor:__________
Change in PIE Factor: (Previous-Current):_________

References

Advances in neurology. (Vol. 40). New York: Raven Press, 1984.

Barbeau, Dr. A. Study concerning incidence of Parkinson's disease in Canada. Source uncertain.

Gray's anatomy. Philadelphia: Lea & Febriger,: 1977.

Lyons & Petrocelli, Medicine, an illustrated history. New York: Abrams, 1978.

Margotta, R. The story of medicine. New York: Golden, 1968.

Null, C. & Null, S. The complete book of nutrition. New York: Dell, 1981.

Physician's desk reference .(38th ed.). New Jersey: Medical Economics.,

Reuben, David R. Everything you always wanted to know about sex but were afraid to ask. New York: Bantam, 1971.

Sandoz Pharmaceuticals. Path program. 1989

Stedman's shorter medical dictionary. Baltimore: Williams & Wiljeins, 1942.

Taber's cyclopedic medical dictionary. (9th ed.). Philadelphia: F.A. Davis Co

The American Parkinson Disease Association. New York.

The Encyclopaedia Britannica. (12th ed.). Chicago.

The Encyclopaedia Britannica. Chicago, 1955.

The Family Book of Preventive Medicine. New York: Simon & Schuster, 1971.

The Medical Show. Consumer Reports. Washington.

The Random House Dictionary. unabridged. (1st ed.). New York: Random House.

Tanner, C., M.D. Rush college of medicine lecture. 1988.

United Parkinsons Foundation. Chicago, IL.

Drug References

Akineton is a trademark of Knoll Pharmaceutical Co., Whippany, NJ 07981.

Artane is a trademark of Lederle, Division of American Cyanamid Co., One Cyanamid Plaza, Wayne, NJ 07470.

Benadryl is a trademark of Parke-Davis, Division of Warner-Lambert, Morris Plains, NJ 07950.

Cogentin is a trademark of Merck, Sharp & Dohme, Division of Merck & Co. Inc., West Point, PA 19486.

Compazine is a trademark of Smith Kline & French Laboratories, Division of Smith Kline Beckman Corp., 1500 Spring Garden St., Philadelphia, PA 19107.

Dopar is a trademark of Norwich Eaton Pharmaceuticals, Norwich, NY 13815.

Kemadrin is a trademark of Burroughs Wellcome Co., 3030 Cornwallis Road, Research Triangle Park, NC 27709.

Larodopa is a trademark of Roche Laboratories, Division of Hoffman-LaRoche Nutley, NJ 07110.

Norflex is a trademark of Riker, subsidiary of 3M Co., 19901 Nordhoff St. Box 1, Northidge, CA 91328.

Norgesic is a trademark of Riker.

Parlodel is a trademark of Sandoz Pharmaceuticals, Division of Sandoz Inc., Rt. 10, West Hanover, NJ 07936.

Parsidol is a trademark of Parke-Davis.

Resperine is a trademark of Henry Suhein Inc., 5 Harbor Park Drive, Port Washington, NY 11050.

Sinemet is a trademark of Merck, Sharp & Dohme.

Thorazine is a trademark of Smith Kline & French.

Tremin is a trademark of Schering Corp., Galloping Hills Road, Kenilworth Hills, NJ 07033.

GLOSSARY

Accouterments: All the material necessary to perform a task.

Acetylcholine: A neuro-transmitter found in the brain, is important to memory process, believed by some to be antagonistic to dopamine.

Acupuncture: A method, chiefly oriental, which treats various ailments by inserting needles into various parts of the body. There is no evidence that it benefits P/D.

Agitation: A shaken emotional state evidenced by erratic facial expressions and uncoordinated body movements indicating inner conflicts. Usually short lived but may require treatment.

Agonist: A chemical which, in P/D, increases or augments neurotransmitter activity. One type (direct acting) is Bromocryptine sold as Parlodel. An indirect acting type is Amantadine sold as Symmetrel. (Not to be confused with antagonist.)

Akinesis: Loss of movement. (See Kinesia.)

Ambidextrous: The ability to use both hands equally well.

Analogue: A term of comparison, for similarities of conditions or things.

Analogy: A comparison of ideas or things citing the similarities rather than the differences.

Animal model: The ability to artificially create in the laboratory a replica of human disease for research purposes.

Anticholinergic: A drug such as Artane or Cogentin which is believed to benefit P/D by acting to neutralize the neuro- transmitter acetylcholine, which is believed by some to be antagonistic to dopamine in the brain.

Antidepressant: One of many drugs referred to as tranquilizers, sometimes prescribed for P/D patients to help control depression, relieve insomnia.

Antihistamine: A family of drugs with many applications as a sedative or relief of symptoms of some allergies and colds. In P/D, Benadryl is useful in reducing tremor.

Antagonist: A chemical which, in P/D, acts to reduce the effectiveness of neuro-transmitters. (Not to be confused with agonist.)

Arthritis, traumatic: An arthritic condition of a joint caused by and following an injury such as a fracture.

Artane: An anticholinergic drug (also sold as Tremin) which chiefly reduces tremor in P/D but is not very effective for other symptoms such as akinesia. Manufactured by Lederle, a division of American Cyanamid Co.

Ataxia: Motor (movement) irregularity or uncoordination in which movements are imprecise and irregular.

Attorney, Power of: A legal document which conveys to another person, usually a spouse or relative, but may be unrelated, the power and authority to act legally on the behalf of the principal or grantor. A Durable Power of Attorney is most often desirable. (See your attorney.)

Autoerotism: Any of a number of activities, mental and physical, which provide sexual arousal and gratification, usually, but not always, by means of masturbation.

Autopsy, brain: Examination of the human brain after death under laboratory conditions. Presently, the only positive confirmation of the diagnosis of P/D.

Benadryl: Trade name for an antihistamine drug diphenhydramine used in P/D to relieve tremor. Manufactured by Parke-Davis.

Bilateral: Physical condition in which both sides of the body behave equally.

Biofeedback: A form of self control of the mind which can be learned, and which can reduce agitation and tension and relieve headaches. Similar to meditation but achieved with electronic devices.

Blink-rate: The frequency with which the reflex momentary closing of the eyelid takes place stated in times per minute. A normal rate may be 10 to 30; for the Parkinsonian it may be 0 to 5. Slow rate may lead to dry eyes requiring eye-drops for lubrication.

Bradykinesis: Extremely slow movement of body and extremities. Common in P/D.

Bradyphrenia: Slowing of thought processes due to diseases, P/D and others.

Brain autopsy: See Autopsy, brain.

Bruxism: Grinding of teeth and clenching of jaw muscles, chiefly involuntary which may take place while awake or asleep. A common symptom of P/D.

Buccinator: A muscle of the face and cheek (the trumpeter's muscle). Loss of effective use contributes to symptoms of P/D including lack of expression, speech problems and drooling.

Cap, childproof: Federal regulations require caps on prescription medicines which are called "childproof" and which are difficult for many adults to open. P/D patients can get their medicines in conventional, easy-to-open containers at no additional cost by requesting them at the pharmacy.

Carbidopa: A drug used for P/D chiefly in combination with Levodopa (in Sinimet). Carbidopa acts to shield Levodopa from destructive enzymes in the body allowing more medication to reach its destination in the brain in the form of dopamine.

Carbon Dioxide: CO2. A normal by-product of respiration. Some research has indicated that in concentration it causes Parkinson's disease- type symptoms. The studies, so far, have been inconclusive.

Carbon Monoxide: CO. A highly toxic by-product of combustion thought by some researchers to be linked with P/D. Studies to date have been inconclusive.

Cardiologist: A physician specializing in diseases of the heart. Sometimes provides clues leading to the diagnosis of P/D through anomalies in EKG's and other symptoms.

Charcot, Jean-Martin: A French neurologist, teacher, experimenter and innovator who lived from 1825-1893. He developed regional criteria and experimented with botanical products in the treatment of Parkinson's disease.

Chemopallidectomy: A stereotaxic surgical procedure, rarely used today, which involved injecting alcohol into a portion of the brain called the Globus Pallidus to stop tremors connected with P/D. Relieved tremor somewhat but caused paralysis instead.

Chiasma: An intersection or crossing point, usually referring to the optic nerves of the eye.

Clitorism: The female equivalent of Priapism. An erection of the clitoris independent of sexual arousal, occasionally reported as a side effect of L-Dopa.

Cogentin: Trade name for benztropine, a drug in the anticholinergic group used in treatment of symptoms of Parkinson's disease. Manufactured by Merck, Sharp & Dohme.

Cramps: Contractions, occasionally violent, of muscles in the lower extremities chiefly. May be related to P/D by way of postural changes or of side effects of prescribed medication.

DATATOP: A research program initiated by private research groups with financial assistance from the NIH. Over a five-year period will do a double-blind study of Deprenyl and Tocopherol in treatment of Parkinson's disease.

Decussation: An intersection or X-shaped crossing point.

Delusions: A mental condition in which the patient has lost touch with reality and has a false conception of what is real and what is illusionary. May be the result of drugs used improperly or may be idiopathic.

Demerol: Trade name for Meperdine, a sedative and analgesic. It has a place in a discussion of P/D only because it was the drug that the illicit laboratory was attempting to synthesize when the MPTP disaster took place. MPTP caused a number of cases of P/D. Demerol is a controlled substance.

Deprenyl: A drug, presently experimental in the United States, which is classified as a dopamine agonist.

Depression: A mental state, not to be confused with being depressed. Depression is a medical problem which involves a negative viewpoint, a lack of self-esteem or hopelessness, usually requiring professional help and medication for recovery.

Dexter: Referring to the right side. Left side is sinister.

Diaphragm: The muscular membrane which separates the abdominal and thoracic cavities of the trunk. Loss of elasticity and distrubed respiration reflexes can cause digestive and respiratory problems for Parkinsonians.

Dominant hemisphere: The central nervous system is bilateral or two-sided. The brain is divided into two hemispheres, each half sending nerve impulses to half of the body, usually the opposite half. Most individuals have a left-dominant brain which makes them right-handed. A right-dominant brain usually makes an individual left-handed.

Dopamine: One of many neuro-transmitters and the principal one in the brain governing motor functions. It occurs naturally in the brain and in other organs. A lack of dopamine causes P/D. The symptoms of P/D are relieved through the use of drugs rich in dopamine such as L-Dopa.

Doppleganger: A shadow or alter ego. A double.

Dyskinesia: Erratic, disorganized, involuntary or unintentional motor movements.

Encephalitis Lethargica: A viral disease wide-spread after the influenza pandemic of 1918. It produced Parkinsonian-like symptoms and at one time was thought to be the cause of P/D.

Eructation: The release of gaseous contents of the stomach by way of the mouth. A belch.

Euphoria: A feeling of well-being or elation. In some circumstances may indicate mental or emotional problems, may be drug related.

Excretory: The process of eliminating waste products from the body by voiding feces and urine.

Eye, Blink-rate: See Blink-rate, eye.

Festination: A condition which develops in P/D among other diseases and is characterized by involuntary hurrying of the walking gait with progressively shortened steps with a tendency for the body to get ahead of the feet.

Flatus: A bubble or accumulation of gas in the intestinal tract, expelled through flatulence or eructation.

Glaucoma: A disease of the eye characterized by increased pressure in the eye which, if neglected, can result in damage to the optic nerve and possibly blindness. Parkinsonians with one type of glaucoma (narrow-angle) are at risk if taking Sinimet.

Globus Pallidus: A portion of the brain once the target of surgery for relief of symptoms of P/D. (See Chemopallidectomy.)

Gross movements: Movement of muscles in large scope or range as compared to microkinesis or minute movements.

Hallucinations: A medical condition, sometimes triggered by medication in which the patient loses touch with reality and sees (or hears, feels or smells) imagined persons or events. Sometimes a side effect of medication prescribed for Parkinson's disease.

Hemisphere, dominant: See Dominant hemisphere.

Immobility: As referred to P/D, indicates an inability to initiate movement. Usually referred to as "freezing".

Impulse, motor: A signal or electrical impulse sent by the brain to a muscle telling the muscle to initiate a movement. In P/D there is a loss of a considerable number of motor impulses.

Incontinence, bladder: The involuntary voiding of urine at places and times not chosen by the patient. Usually indicates disturbance of the urinary sphincter in P/D. (See a urologist.)

Incontinence, bowel: Involuntary flatulence and voiding of feces at times and places not chosen by the patient. Usually indicates disturbance of the anal sphincter in P/D.

Kinesia: More properly, kinetics. Deals with motion.

L-Dopa: The first chemical product to relieve symptoms of P/D by supplementing the naturally occurring dopamine in the brain. L-dopa is in its third and fourth generations and is much improved as to effectiveness and reduced side-effects. It is commonly sold as Sinimet, combining Carbidopa and Levodopa.

Linguistics: The science of language, the study of how we speak and why we speak as we do. May be beneficial to the P/D patient on two levels: (1) Basic research to determine the mechanics of speech and their interrelation with, and function of the two hemispheres of the brain; and, (2) Assistance for the P/D patient in improving and preserving his speech.

Living Will: A legal document by means of which an individual can, for whatever good reasons, prior to its being needed, leave specific directions for his doctors not to take any heroic measures such as surgery to prolong his life after it has been determined that no recovery is possible. Most states have a Living Will, or Right to Die, law but are strict about form and provisions. (See your attorney.)

Mobility: The ability to move about under one's own power. Ambulatory.

Motor Impulse: See impulse, motor.

Movement, gross: See Gross movement.

MPPP: A designer drug, made illegally which mimics the effect of Demerol, a controlled substance.

MPTP: A chemical produced by accident in an attempt to produce MPPP. MPTP attacks the brain producing an advanced case of P/D in a matter of days. This chemical has enabled research scientists to produce an animal model of P/D in the laboratory, one of the most significant events in Parkinson's disease research since the introduction of L-Dopa.

Neuroleptic: A family of drugs prescribed for a number of conditions not related to P/D. Neuroleptics are known to be dopamine antagonists which can make the symptoms of P/D worse. Common neuroleptica are Compazine and Thorazine.

Neuro-transmitter: A family of chemical compounds which occur normally in the body and act to facilitate passage of nerve impulses. Examples are dopamine, acetylcholine and GABA. Several neurotransmitters are antagonistic to each other and must be prescribed with care.

Night horrors: Pavor Nocturnis. An extremely disturbing dream involving anxiety and very real images of the dreamer and his loved ones.

Nightmares: Dreams of a disturbing nature involving anxiety and sometimes feelings of suffocation.

Nocturnal: Taking place at night.

On-off syndrome: The pronounced switching "on" or "off" effect noticed by almost all P/D patients when medication takes effect or wears off. This effect is the object of much study hoping to smooth out the hills and valleys, and a timed-release Sinimet is soon to be released.

Orbicularis Oculi: Muscle(s) in the orbit of the eye. An example of the smaller muscles of the body which may be affected by P/D.

Orthopedist: A medical doctor specializing in the treatment of skeletal and muscular structures of the body.

Palsy: The loss of control and use of a muscle or group of muscles. May be due to P/D or other causes.

Pain: A condition in which a patient feels discomfort of varying locale, intensity and duration. Pain is not usually a factor or a component in the symptoms of P/D.

Palsy, shaking: An archaic term for P/D.

Paralysis, agitans: A term formerly applied to P/D, now little used.

Parkinsonian: For purposes of this text, referring to a person who has been diagnosed and is being treated as a Parkinson's disease patient.

Parkinsonism: A neurological disorder which meets the criteria for Parkinson's disease: resting tremor, slow movements, postural instability and loss of joint flexibility.

Parkinson's disease, drug-induced:

A type of Parkinsonism which is caused by identifiable drugs, often members of the neuroleptic family (Thorazine, Compazine or Resperine) and which are reversible. (This category does not include the MPTP-designer-drug-produced Parkinson's disease which is a near perfect analogue to P/D and which is believed irreversible.)

Parkinson's disease, encephalitic: Parkinson's disease with the diagnosis meeting all the tests for P/D but in a patient with a history of Encephalitis.

Parkinson's disease, idiopathic: A neurological disorder which meets all of the criteria for Parkinson's disease but for which no cause has been determined.

Parkinson's Syndrome: A neurological manifestation in which symptoms associated with P/D are present but which cannot be reliably diagnosed as Parkinson's disease.

Parlodel: Bromocryptine Mesylate. Sold as Parlodel by Sandoz Inc. Parlodel is a direct acting agonist which acts to stimulate dopamine receptors directly.

Paroxysm, anal: A spasm or sudden discomfort of the anal sphincter. In P/D, often related to bowel incontinence.

Paroxysm, bladder: A spasm or sudden discomfort in the bladder sphincter. In P/D, often related to bladder incontinence.

Perambulation: The act of moving about on one's own, freely and with relative ease.

Peristalsis: The wave-like sequential contractions of muscles in the esophagus and in the intestinal tract by means of which ingested food is moved through these bodies.

Perspicacity: The ability to see or understand a complex concept readily.

Pill-Rolling: A type of palsy seen in P/D, so called because the motion of the hand and forearm which mimics rolling a pill between the thumb and finger.

Power of Attorney: See Attorney, Power of.

Priapism: In the male, an erection of the penis without stimulus or sexual arousal. Sometimes seen as a side-effect of L-Dopa. Female equivalent is clitorism.

Psychiatrist: A medical doctor with the special training required to diagnose and treat mental and emotional disorders. Sometimes is a consultant on mental problems associated with P/D: depression, hallucinations and dementia.

Quadriceps: A large muscle in the front of the thigh, one of the largest in the body.

Radiologist: A medical doctor trained in the use and interpretation of X-rays and other imaging techniques primarily in the diagnosis of medical problems.

Reflex, knee-jerk: The reflex contraction of muscles of the leg when struck with a mallet just below the kneecap. Normally quite strong and bilaterally uniform in healthy individuals. The reflex may be diminished or of a different character in the two legs. The knee-jerk is useful to a neurologist in making a diagnosis of P/D and isolating other diseases with similar symptoms.

Reflex, startle: A reflex action when the patient involuntarily, with his extremities or his whole body, draws away from a sound or a touch he is not expecting.

Resting tremor: One of the more common symptoms of P/D in which tremor is more pronounced at rest than when in motion. A tremor in an extremity while in motion can be due to many other ailments not related to P/D.

Salivation: The production of saliva in the mouth of Parkinsonians sometimes seems excessive and is compounded by disturbance of the normal swallow reflex. The loss of muscle tone and motor impulses can result in drooling as the disease worsens.

Sinequan: A mild sedative and tranquilizer, often prescribed for Parkinsonians as an aid to sleep.

Sinister: Left-side or left-hand preference. (See Dexter.)

Spasm: A condition in which a muscle or group of muscles involuntarily contracts. May affect smooth or striated muscles. A sustained spasm is called a cramp.

Sphincter: A muscle or group of muscles, ring shaped, which close off or regulate the size of an opening. Examples are the pyloric between the stomach and the duodenum; the bladder sphincter; and an external and an internal in the anus. Their ability to control is gradually lost or diminished as P/D grows worse.

Spontaneous: Taking place without a specific action or stimulus.

Stereotaxic surgery: When in reference to the brain, represents direct contact with the brain by some foreign agent, a surgical tool or instrument, such as a cryogenic probe. Chemopallidectomy, for example.

Stimuli: Pleural of stimulus. A goad or incitement to cause some sort of action. A trigger.

Symmetrel: A trade name for Amantadene which is prescribed to supplement other medicines prescribed for P/D. Manufactured by DuPont Pharmaceuticals.

Tocopherol: A drug being studied for its possible benefit to P/D in a double-blind format in the DATATOP program.

Traumatic Arthritis: See Arthritis, traumatic.

Tremor: An involuntary movement of parts of the body triggered by alternately contracting opposing muscles as in Parkinson's disease.

Tremor, resting: See Resting tremor.

Will: A legal document stating the intended disposition of one's estate after one's death.

Will, Living: See Living Will.

Index

A

Alcohol consumption, 13-94
Animal Model, 1-11
Autopsy
 Request for, 6-34

B

Belladona, 1-9
Biofeedback devices, 11-67
Blink-rate
 Effect on, 4-23
Blood pressure, 13-89
Bruxism, 5-31

C

Caregiver
 As a team with the patient, 15-112
 Attitudes and motivations, Intro-3
 Dcfinition, Intro-3
Charcot, Jean
 P/D research, 1-9
Constipation, 13-95
 Treatment of, 12-76
Cramps, 13-90

D

Dental problems, 13-88
Depression
 Definition of, 9-48
 Medications to treat, 9-48
 Treatment for, 8-43
 Ways of avoiding, 9-49
Dexterity, loss of
 Compensations for, 13-81
Digestive disorders
 Constipation, 12-76
 Excretion of feces, 12-75
 Increase of intestinal gas, 12-75
Doctor-patient relationship, 4-25
 Advance preparations for visit, 5-28
Dopamine, 1-10
Driving, 13-96
 Changing the pace, 13-97
 Giving up, 13-96
 Special parking spaces, 13-97

E

Evaluation scales
 H & Y, 1-12
 Personal method, 1-13
 URSP, 1-12
Exercise
 Delaying muscle deterioration, 5-30
 For flexibility, 14-101
 For strength, 14-107
 Pacing yourself, 14-102

F

Falls
 As a result of festination, 10-55
 Causes of, 10-55
 Due to lowered blood pressure, 10-56
 Reducing the incidences of, 10-56
Family physician
 Diagnosis and treatment of P/D, 4-22
Flexibility exercises, 14-103

H

Hallucinations
 Drug-induced, 9-50
Hypotension
 Drug-related, 13-89

I

Incontinence, 5-31
 Digestive disorders, 12-75
 Excretory problems, 12-74
 Urinary problems, 12-74
 Use of absorbent undergarments, 12-76

K

Kinesia
 Relation to P/D, Intro-5

L

L-Dopa
 Dopamine substitute, 1-10
L-Dopa therapy
 Effect on sex live, 12-73
Living Will
 Preparation of, 6-34
Local support groups, 15-111
 And the lone Parkinsonian, 15-111
 Problems in organizing/sustaining, 15-113

M

Manual tasks
 Loss of dexterity, 13-80
 Loss of legible handwritting, 13-81
Medication
 For use in treating depression, 9-48
 Relief of symptoms, 6-32
 Side effects of, 5-29
Mental attitudes
 Effects from physical activity, 10-56
Mobility problems
 Acrotaxia, 4-25
 Festination, 4-24
 Tendency to fall, 4-24
MPPP, 7-39
MPTP, 1-12

N

National organizations, 15-110
 Addresses for, 15-114
Neurologist
 Treatment of P/D, 4-21
Nutrition
 Food cures for P/D, 13-92
 Studies concerning L-Dopa, 13-93

P

Parkinson's disease
 Among the elderly, 2-15
 Breakthroughs in research, 7-37
 Definition, 1-7
 Dental problems, 13-88
 Diagnosis of, 4-21
 Effects of exercise, 14-101
 Effects on driving, 13-96
 Effects on eyesight, 13-82
 Encephalitis connection, 1-9
 Evaluation scales, 1-12
 Fears and life expectancy, 2-17
 Incidence and symptoms, 1-8
 Local support groups, 15-111
 Loss of brain cells, 9-47
 Maintaining ambulatory stages, 13-79

Mobility problems, 4-24
National organizations, 15-110
Nutrition, 13-91
Psychological problems, 8-42
Research findings, 2-15
Surgical procedures, 1-10
Tell-tale signs, 4-23
Terminology, Intro-4
Time as an ally, 7-36
Parkinson's Syndrome, Intro-5
73 Parkinson, Dr. James, 1-8
Parkinsonian
Definition, Intro-5
Parkinsonism, Intro-5
drug-induced, Intro-5
Perambulation, 13-77
Controlling inertia, 13-78
Festination, 13-78
Ploys for moving about, 13-77
Physiological problems, 10-54
Climbing/descending steps, 13-79
Coping with, 11-60
Excretory problems, 12-69
Fatigue, 10-57
Festination, 10-55
Lowered blood pressure, 10-56
Pain and P/D, 10-58
Progression of, 10-55
Sexual dysfunction, 12-69
Sleeping arrangements, 11-65
Swallowing, breathing and speech difficulties, 13-84
Threat of falls, 10-55
Power of Attorney, 6-34
Psychological problems
Altered self-image, 8-42
Avoiding negative attitudes, 9-51
Depression, 8-43
Importance of mental challenges, 8-44
More serious problems, 8-45
Recognizing and evaluating, 9-46

R

Research breakthroughs
Medications, 7-37
MPTP animal model, 7-37
Pump-implant project, 7-38
Surgical procedures, 7-40
Resting tremor
Effects from surgery, 1-10

S

Salivation dysfunction, 4-23
Bruxism, 4-23
Sexual concerns
Adjustments in techniques/habits, 12-70
Autoerotism, 12-71
Need for communication, 12-70
Seeking professional counsel, 12-73
Sex drive, 12-70
Typical problems among females, 12-71
Typical problems among males, 12-71
Use of masturbation, 12-72
Use of pornography, 12-72
73 Shock therapy
Use of in treatment for depression, 8-44
Sleeping arrangements, 11-65
Sheets, pillows, etc., 11-65
Use of a sleep mask, 11-66
Smoking, 13-94
Speech difficulties, 4-24
Cause of, 13-85
Loss of volume and intelligibility, 5-31
Speech therapy
Need for, 13-86
Strength exercises, 14-107

Equipment for, 14-107
Terminology, 14-107
Surgical procedures
Cell-implant, 7-40
Swallowing dysfunctions
Choking, 13-87
Heimlich Maneuver, 13-87
Salivation problems, 13-88
Symptoms, 1-8
Bilateral or unilateral, 5-30
Cramps, 9-50
Loss of dexterity, 5-30
Sleep disturbances, 9-50
Susceptibility to hot and cold, 4-25

T

Treatment
Ruling out other diseases, 4-22

U

Urinary problems
Need for medical attention, 12-74
Sudden urge to urinate, 12-75

V

Visual problems
Attributing to P/D, 13-83
Need to see an ophthalmologist, 13-83
Symptoms, 13-83

W

Will
Need for, 6-34